D1206772

Uncorrected Galleys

Uncorrected Galleys

Stolen Motherhood

Uncorrected Galleys

Uncorrected Galleys

Maria De Koninck

Stolen Motherhood
Surrogacy and Made-to-Order Children

Translated by Arielle Aaronson

Baraka
Books

Montréal

Uncorrected Galleys

All rights reserved. No part of this book may be reproduced or transmitted in any form or by any means, electronic or mechanical, including photocopying, recording, or by any information storage and retrieval system, without permission in writing from the publisher.

© Baraka Books
Translation © Arielle Aaronson

ISBN 978-1-77186-224-0 pbk; 978-1-77186-233-2 epub; 978-1-77186-234-9 pdf

Cover design by Maison 1608
Book Design by Folio infographie
Proofreading by Rachel Hewitt, Robin Philpot

Legal Deposit, 3rd quarter 2020
Bibliothèque et Archives nationales du Québec
Library and Archives Canada

Published by Baraka Books of Montreal

Printed and bound in Quebec

TRADE DISTRIBUTION & RETURNS
Canada – UTP Distribution: UTPdistribution.com

UNITED STATES
Independent Publishers Group: IPGbook.com

We acknowledge the support, including translation support, from the Société de développement des entreprises culturelles (SODEC) and the Government of Quebec tax credit for book publishing administered by SODEC.

Société
de développement
des entreprises
culturelles
Québec

Funded by the Government of Canada
Financé par le gouvernement du Canada | Canada

To all the women who, in the course of research I have participated in, have generously agreed to share their experience of maternity.

Uncorrected Galleys

Uncorrected Galleys

Contents

Uncorrected Galleys

Uncorrected Galleys

Foreword

The first successful in vitro fertilization took place just over forty years ago—the blink of an eye in the history of humanity. Yet this technique has made such rapid advances that today, it enables individuals or couples hoping to reproduce to have recourse to a third person for the duration of a pregnancy.

Using surrogate mothers is no longer a marginal practice, nor does it take place in secrecy; it is a growing phenomenon, though there has been no informed debate on the potential social impacts of its trivialization as a means of reproductive intervention.[1] Nevertheless, in our society and elsewhere, discourse has evolved to normalize surrogacy, even touting it as social progress. This discourse is structured to discredit those who question the practice, painting them as resistant to change and progress, blind to today's realities.

To be truly modern, a society should rely on knowledge acquired from the social sciences (sociology, anthropology, economics, psychology), philosophy, law, medicine, psychiatry, and neuroscience, among other

Uncorrected Galleys

fields, to examine advancements in surrogacy, grasp its components, and evaluate its consequences.

What exactly is the "surrogacy process"? It is a way to permit people to reproduce by commissioning a woman to carry a child and requiring her to surrender it to someone else after giving birth. In most cases, she withdraws from the child's life completely. This method represents a fundamental change in our understanding and experience of reproduction, since it cannot be likened to other customs of child circulation observed in so-called traditional societies, as we will discuss later on.

Surrogacy is not a biomedical advance independent of social relationships. In challenging the definition of motherhood by dividing and sharing it between different women, surrogacy acts on the meaning of motherhood as a feminine experience. This is why contemplating the meaning of this process in reference to the experience of motherhood forces a broader reflection on the nature of gender relations, the meaning of human reproduction, and the status of the child within the society into which it is born.

Only humans can envision a future; they are the only beings that are conscious of their mortality. It follows that they are also the only beings to give meaning to the possibility of prolonging their memory through children. This extension, recognized socially as filiation, is defined and framed across all societies. As cultural constructs, definitions and frameworks differ from one society to another.

In nature, reproduction happens when two people come together and create a unique third: a profound experience of otherness. Yet once the child is born, the transmission of knowledge, culture, or belonging within a social group is not always performed by these two biological parents. Various traditions or events can account for why, after birth, a child may be entrusted to others who will educate it and serve as family—one that does not include the natural parents.

Who is my mother? Who is my father? Who are my grandparents, sisters, brothers, and the members of my extended family? These are universal human markers, points of reference that, ideally, everyone should have. They enable an individual to forge an identity, and their absence presents a path often riddled with obstacles, as evidenced by the efforts of adopted children to find their biological parents. Accounts of children who are adopted into loving families, but who nevertheless wish to meet their biological parents, confirm the complexity of developing an identity. Several such accounts were heard in Quebec in 2017 during the debate on the Act to amend the Civil Code and other legislative provisions concerning adoption and the disclosure of information.[2]

Until recently, human reproduction was never considered to be a matter of technique or process. It has only become so with the advent of medically assisted procreation, also called assisted human reproduction (AHP), and especially with the use of surrogate mothers, which introduces a new element when it comes to designating caretakers for the newborn child. This process involves an arrangement prior to conception that names someone other than the birth mother to be responsible for the child. The surrogate knows, even before carrying the child, that she will not take care of it once it is born and, contrary to what has been observed in so-called traditional societies, commits to this not in a communal context, but rather in a context defined by the exercise of individual freedoms.

Wanting to procreate is a natural human desire. It ensures the survival of the species and, on an individual level, can be seen as a way to extend oneself and carry one's legacy forward. The egocentric aspect of reproduction may be one factor in the desire to self-perpetuate through a child, but it is far from the only one. Furthermore, the scope of this aspect varies greatly between cultures.

In some environments, even today, procreating is a social duty: it is an expectation primarily aimed at women through the implementation of social controls, including potential penalties for those who fail to conform. In others, procreating is an individual choice. Similarly, the responsibility of caring for a child can be assumed or supported by a community or can be essentially entrusted to the parents.

Human reproduction cannot be discussed without taking into account a set of psychological, social, cultural, and economic factors, among others. These raise issues that deserve consideration if we want to understand how surrogacy practices evolve.

This essay aims to define, as much as possible, how normalizing surrogacy might transform human relations, including gender relations, by jeopardizing human dignity—a defining principle of social organization.

It certainly isn't my goal to cover all of these aspects. Yet I feel it is important to speak out now about commissioning women to carry children according to prior arrangements requiring them to surrender their children to the commissioning parents and renounce motherhood. Much of the reflection and research underpinning my arguments is empirical. Studies concerned with family planning, pregnancy, childbirth, and motherhood have helped me document these different experiences here and elsewhere. I consider this my duty on behalf of all the women who have recounted their experiences of motherhood over the years, as part of various studies I have either led or participated in. I cannot remain silent when faced with the absence of sound debate, attempts to tarnish sentiments as noble as altruism, efforts to appropriate women under the guise of progress, and lack of regard for children's wellbeing. I believe it is crucial to speak out, to offer a vision that is different from the one centred on the needs of individuals and couples who wish to become parents within a context where the proposed "solution" has not been analyzed from the point of view of its human and social

Uncorrected Galleys

consequences. My focus is largely on motherhood and the children's future.

Drawing on knowledge acquired across several disciplines, I consider the issue from three angles: the feminist angle, including an analysis of surrogacy and its development in the context of gender relations; the sociological angle, in the context of human rights and our lives within society; and the ethical angle, that of a system of shared values—many of which are upheld by laws, charters, and regulations—and more specifically, that of respect for human dignity.

Introduction

Surrogacy is based on an agreement between a woman who undertakes to carry and bear a child, and one or two individuals to whom she will surrender the child so they can become the parent or parents. Most often they are referred to as "intended parents," a term coined in the United States that defines parents based on their intention to have a child. But the concept of intention is purely theoretical. An *intention* is a desire to accomplish something—in this case, a have a child—which is not the same as a concrete fact.

In the case of contractual procreation, individuals with such a desire enter into an arrangement with a third person, a woman, which effectively allows them to "commission" a child. They undertake to become the child's parents and assume all related responsibilities. In return, they cover the costs incurred by this person or pay her for the pregnancy. This nuance of an "intention"-turned-commission is significant, since the underlying issue involves planning for a birth in contractual terms.

The process of surrogacy can take on a variety of forms, depending on the circumstances and the terms of the arrangement. In most cases, commissioning parents have no relationship to the mother. But sometimes they are friends, or even family. The latter case raises preoccupations, some of which concern the prohibition of incest (symbolic or "type two").[1] Can a woman carry her brother's child if her sister-in-law is unable to? Can a grandmother act as surrogate on behalf of her son or daughter?

The question of incest must be addressed. Incest is a universal benchmark in defining family ties. According to Spanish anthropologist Enric Porqueres i Gené, director of the School for Advanced Studies in the Social Sciences in Paris, ethnological studies demonstrate that the association of corporeity and kinship "lies at the core of all kinship systems." Gené writes that the "strength of this association [between corporeity and kinship] is particularly clear when it comes to incest prohibitions," which he considers "the least common denominator of kinship systems."[2] The risk of incest is now raised with the use of reproductive technologies (especially gamete donation), associated with anonymity and therefore a lack of information. Children born from ova or sperm donations (most often anonymous), unaware that they were created by gametes of the same people, may risk engaging in incestuous relationships. In cases of surrogacy, the question of incest is not raised according to the usual criteria, but it is raised nonetheless. These concerns are a reminder that reproduction is anchored in the body, even if discourses promoting assisted reproduction tend to disembody it.

Sometimes the mother does remain in the child's family circle, though these cases are rare. In the early days of the practice, the surrogate mother would have been inseminated with the father's sperm. Today, she usually receives an embryo following in vitro fertilization with another woman's ovum—in some situations this is the father's spouse, in which case the commissioning couple provides both gametes.

The pregnancy and transfer of the child can be free, meaning there is no remuneration involved. This is generally referred to as *altruistic* surrogacy, the woman being only compensated for fees incurred throughout the pregnancy. But other arrangements exist, too. Some people live in areas where surrogacy is prohibited, or they simply don't have access to a surrogate willing to carry a child for free; others prefer to deal with a stranger. In these cases, they often turn to places where *commercial* (paid) surrogacy is allowed, many of which are low-income countries.

There is no fixed price for surrogacy. Costs can be quite high, as is sometimes the case in the United States, or very low, such as in Asia or Africa. The fees paid to intermediaries, who establish contact between the commissioning parents and surrogates and also take care of all or part of the necessary arrangements

Uncorrected Galleys

(contract, prenatal care, delivery fees, etc.), are generally high and represent a significant part of the total cost.[3] The more women come from underprivileged backgrounds and countries offering little social protection, the less they are paid. For that reason, questioning surrogacy often comes with the argument that it is a shameless exploitation of women living in low-income areas for whom commercial pregnancy is a way to improve their personal and their family's condition. These women agree to such an arrangement since the payout is much higher than what they would earn from working. We will return to this issue later.

Legality in Quebec and Canada

In Quebec, according to article 541 of the Civil Code, "Any agreement whereby a woman undertakes to procreate or carry a child for another person is absolutely null."[4] This means that surrogacy arrangements between a woman and one or more commissioning parents are not legally recognized. In Canada, the 2004 Assisted Human Reproduction Act (AHRA) stipulates that the procedure must be done without compensation.[5] It defines a surrogate as a "female person who—with the intention of surrendering the child at birth to a donor or another person—carries an embryo or foetus that was conceived by means of an assisted reproduction procedure and derived from the genes of a donor or donors,"[6] and specifies that the surrogate must be at least twenty-one.[7] It states: "No person shall pay consideration to a female person to be a surrogate mother, offer to pay such consideration or advertise that it will be paid."[8]

This also concerns intermediaries, since it is prohibited to "accept consideration for arranging for the services of a surrogate mother, offer to make an arrangement for such consideration or advertise the arranging of such services,"[9] and no person "shall pay consideration to another person to arrange for the services of a surrogate mother, offer to pay such consideration or advertise the payment of it." [10]

In 2019, Health Canada announced that section 12 of the AHRA would come into force on June 9, 2020, along with the *Reimbursement Related to Assisted Human Reproduction Regulations*. This provides for the reimbursement of expenditures incurred by surrogate mothers (and ova or sperm donors). Between 2017 and 2019 Health Canada conducted consultations, including one with the assisted reproduction "industry," in order to define what fees should be included in the regulations.[11]

Commercial surrogacy is currently prohibited in Canada. Nevertheless, it is openly used by many Canadians. President of the Treasury Board Scott Brison (2016-2019) and his partner bought ova and hired the "services" of a surrogate in the United States for a hefty sum.[12] That this fact doesn't appear to trouble members of government should surprise. And yet, even the Global Affairs Canada website offers advice for "Canadians considering entering into a surrogacy arrangement."[13] What is illegal in Canada is legal elsewhere. According to the government, Canadians can therefore go elsewhere. On May 29, 2018, Liberal backbencher Anthony Housefather introduced a private member's bill, an *"Act to amend the Assisted Human Reproduction Act,"* to decriminalize the practice of compensating surrogate mothers as well as ova and sperm donors. In November of the same year, he announced that the bill would not be submitted to Parliament before the federal elections scheduled for October 2019.[14]

Alongside the "market" for surrogates and their "donations" is the market for ova. It is becoming more common for commissioning parents to obtain ova, preferring the surrogate mother not also be the "genetic mother" of the unborn child. But there are rules for this, too. Canada prohibits individuals from purchasing either sperm or ova (article 7[1] of the AHRA). Yet this doesn't seem to prevent companies from acting as intermediaries and presenting a catalogue of their egg donors, including information on their personal characteristics.[15]

Here is the response to a complaint I filed with Health Canada in June 2018 against Can-Am Cryoservices, whose operations are a priori illegal:

> According to the *Assisted Human Reproduction Act* (AHRA) it is prohibited, among other things, to purchase sperm or ova from a person acting on behalf of a donor, to purchase sperm or ova from a donor, or to advertise

for such a purchase. This means that in Canada, a donor cannot receive compensation in any form (money, gifts, services, etc.) for a sperm or ova donation.

The AHRA does not prohibit the purchase of sperm or ova **from a person other than the donor, provided this person isn't acting on behalf of the donor.**[16] Nor does the AHRA prohibit selling or offering to sell sperm or ova. **This means that the AHRA permits fertility clinics and sperm banks to charge fees for their services, which may include the storage, transfer, and use of donated ova or sperm.** Can-Am Cryoservices is considered an importer and distributor of donor semen intended for assisted reproduction, and is subject to the Processing and Distribution of Semen for Assisted Conception Regulations.[17]

The Canadian government has filed very few lawsuits pursuant to this act, except against the owner of the Canadian Fertility Consulting (CFC) firm. In 2013, CFC was forced to pay a $60,000 fine for violations including remitting money to surrogate mothers—which did nothing to deter the company from continuing its activities, quite the contrary.[18]

Regarding other countries, legal provisions vary greatly, as we will see.

Several ways to name the same practice

Choice of words is never trivial, since words influence our worldview. This is the case for the various terms and expressions that refer to contract motherhood.[19] Here are the terms referred to or used in this essay: gestational carrier, surrogacy, use of surrogate mothers, and third-party reproducers.

Gestational carriers

Gestational carriers is a frequently used term, whereas the concept of "gestation" belongs to the animal world; for humans, the term "pregnancy" is preferred. The word "gestation" puts the emphasis on the physiological aspect of pregnancy and eliminates all reference to motherhood, which is a human experience. This concept distinguishes the so-called gestational carrier from the mother of the child. A report submitted in 2018 to the United Nations Human Rights Council criticizes this designation:

> The legal fiction of the "never-a-mother" gestational carrier is a legal concept which is used to justify denial of the surrogate mother's rights. Once the surrogate mother is reduced, during pregnancy, to a never-a-mother gestational carrier acting for the benefit of intending parents, the door is open to enforcing contracts that purport to alienate her rights and freedoms.[20]

By qualifying the gestator as a carrier, we understand that the goal is to carry the child for someone else. In the case of a gestational carrier, the gestator is generally not biologically related to the child she is carrying.

In order to specify the chosen approach, the term "altruistic" (a concept with roots in humanism[21]) is often added to characterize the practice as a gift rather than a contractual agreement. If remuneration is involved, "commercial" is added, a qualifier that is less shocking when it is associated with "gestation" than "mother," as the latter references a human role with regard to the child.

Surrogacy[22]

This designates the fact of carrying a child for someone else, where the pregnant woman is considered only a substitute and called the "surrogate." "Surrogacy" illustrates the desired distance between the woman and the child she is carrying and to whom she will give birth.

Previously, the practice involved insemination of the surrogate, or "traditional surrogacy"; generally, this is no longer the case. Increasingly, motherhood is being shared between two women: one who supplies the ova and one who receives the embryo transfer (via in vitro techniques), which has been fertilized by the man's sperm in cases of heterosexual commissioning couples, or by one or both of the two men (mixed sperm) in cases of homosexual couples. The use of two women echoes the concept of a gestational carrier, which in some ways separates conception from pregnancy.

Commissioning parents often prefer this fragmentation of motherhood, since it creates distance between the surrogate and the genetically unrelated child and leaves more room for the commissioning parents.

Uncorrected Galleys

Jérôme Courduriès, French anthropologist and professor at Université Toulouse–Jean Jaurès, writes:

> When it comes to surrogacy, dissociating gestation from conception seems to be a way of both diminishing the maternal nature of the surrogate, and reinforcing the pre-eminence of the parent couple in the fulfillment of the parental project.[23]

This method is also less expensive, since it involves enlisting a woman only for the duration of the pregnancy and also disregards her features (e.g., her skin colour). In other words, you can save money by hiring a non-white woman in a low-income country and still end up with a white child!

Use of surrogate mothers

This expression comprises two elements. The first, "use," refers to a demand: we must not forget the practice exists due to a demand. Adding "mothers" to surrogates reminds us that although these women carry children for other people, they experience motherhood during these nine months. To consider them mere "gestators" is something of a delusion, since it discounts the complexity and depth of the experience, along with maternal-foetal exchanges in utero that are scientifically well documented.

Third-party reproduction

This label, particularly prevalent in the English-speaking world, is part of a normalizing discourse surrounding reproduction implicating more than two people, apart from medical staff. To its credit, the concept is very clear. It confers the status of an "outside" actor who facilitates reproduction on the woman who carries and gives birth to the child.

A few definitions: procreation, kinship, descent

Before going further, we must define several other concepts used when describing the process of human reproduction and its frameworks. Their meaning impacts how we understand changes brought about through the use of reproductive techniques that enable surrogacy. These terms refer to human practices that vary among societies and social eras. Knowledge of these practices, or at least some of them, helps us gauge whether they are relevant to discussions around the legitimacy of new practices in our society (i.e., some outcomes of medical intervention are considered comparable to what already exists in so-called traditional societies).

The concept of "procreation" signifies the gift of life. We can think of it as "creating a being other than oneself." Medically assisted procreation refers to the gift of life made possible with the help of medicine. In theory, medicine should not intervene when it comes

Uncorrected Galleys

to the social rules that govern how we recognize social links with children, nor when it comes to our responsibilities towards them. But it is not so simple, since medicine establishes the diagnoses that justify medical assistance for reproduction, and is therefore granted a social power when defining sterility. This power isn't new: many examples illustrate the evolution of diagnoses that have been modulated by social norms. History is rife with cases involving control of women's bodies or behaviours that were considered marginal.

The notion of "kinship" is also debated. Kinship represents a discipline in itself; there are myriad studies on the subject. Anthropological research has improved our understanding of the interpersonal connections by which humans govern certain relationships, including the designation of parents, organization of guardianship, and transmission of knowledge, skills, and goods, among other things. Here is a general definition of kinship: "In anthropology, kinship is the 'blood ties,' the network of socially recognized relationships orbiting the Ego"[24] (the individual around whom kinship relations are defined).[25]

From a legal standpoint, kinship is defined as "the lawful relationship between persons who are descended one from the other or from a common predecessor: father, mother, and children, grandparents and grandchildren, brothers and sisters, cousins, uncles and aunts, nephews and nieces."[26] The Civil Code of Quebec stipulates that "[kinship] is based on ties of blood or of adoption."[27]

Descent, a component of any kinship system[28] and one that is central to the question of surrogacy, is defined in anthropological terms as "a set of rights and obligations conferred on a member of a social group defined by the transmission of lineage positions from one generation to another."[29] Here the term *generation* refers to the genealogical level, or the distance from a common ancestor. The child is generation 0, its parents, generation 1.[30]

Under Quebec law, descent (filiation) is defined as "the family relationship between a child and the child's parents."[31] This link can be established by blood, by assisted reproduction, or by adoption.

Through descent, a child becomes part of a "genealogical space, that of his or her paternal and maternal forbears [...]" and is "connected to the human species, finds his place, and becomes part of a continuity that gives meaning to his life."[32] This is why we must reflect on changes prompted by the use of reproductive technologies and their impact on how children are situated within a lineage.

The term "parenthood" is a relatively recent concept and refers to the assuming of parental duties by a person who is not necessarily legally recognized as such. Its use has grown along with the rise in blended families, among other factors, which are a result of changing views on marriage. However, it also opens new channels for those wanting to take on parental responsibilities and play a role comparable to that of parent without establishing a line of descent.

Uncorrected Galleys

This introduction illustrates just how complex interventions in human reproduction can be. They not only represent new ways of doing things, but can also lead to profound changes in human relations by transforming the connections between individuals who reproduce, as well as their responsibilities towards the resulting children. Moreover, these interventions can alter how a child is inscribed into the lineage of preceding generations.

Chapter 1

Surrogacy's Emergence, Development, and International Expansion

Surrogacy raises many issues and cannot be addressed or discussed without taking into account the social, cultural, and economic factors that underpin it. Nor can surrogacy be compared to pre-existing procedures from which it could be legitimised, since the socio-cultural and economic contexts governing the practice are fundamentally different. It must therefore be examined in today's context while identifying the factors that encouraged its spread.

Changes that prompted the development of reproductive practices

Surrogacy falls within the scope of medically assisted reproduction, which encompasses a number of biomedical interventions. The process begins with ovarian stimulation, followed by artificial insemination or oocyte retrieval. The next step is in vitro fertilization, using sperm provided by the commissioning parent(s), followed by embryo implantation.

Medically assisted reproductive techniques have developed very rapidly since the 1960s, in the wake of an evolution in obstetrics. The end of the 1970s saw a rise in women solicited to bear children that they would be expected to surrender. Why? Quite simply because it had become medically possible.

This situation today is the product of a social evolution. Advances in science are made as questions are raised and experiments allowed and performed.[1] Even once medically assisted reproduction became possible, it would not have been employed or popularized if it had not found a social breeding ground (a justification, a procedure, and a demand).

To understand how surrogacy became possible and later widespread, we must view it through our current social context, underscoring the various social changes that have enabled its proliferation. Quebec and Canada are not cut off from the rest of the world; though they have unique features, they nonetheless fit into a wider context of development observable in other Western nations. Specifically concerned here are the changes regarding the notion of personhood, the status of women, the transformation of the family, the status of children, the evolution of knowledge and discourse, and widespread changes to the global economy. These issues cannot be considered in isolation, nor separated from the evolution of scientific knowledge or reproductive interventions that followed.

Human rights, the individual, and freedom

The notion of the individual, associated with the recognition of human rights, has become a tenet of Western societies. The advancement of individual rights is generally seen as the advancement of human dignity, a core value as well as a legal principle. Yet reality is rarely simple, and limits are not always easy to establish.

Individual rights exist within a social context and may be at odds with other individual rights. When some groups call for certain rights to be recognized, their denial is interpreted as discriminatory—even though exercising these rights may infringe on the rights of other groups. Moreover, the foundations of the claims themselves may not be rooted in recognized rights. In the context of surrogacy, for instance, there is no basis for the "right to child" claim that certain groups defend.[2]

The same goes for individual liberties: respecting human rights means respecting individual liberties, but to what extent? Defining these limits gives rise to major debates, ones that are particularly heated when it comes to reproduction.

This evolution coincided with a surge in individualism, or "the doctrine whereby the value of the individual is intrinsically superior to anything else, in all areas—ethics, politics, economics—where the rights and responsibilities of the latter always prevail."[3]

The status of women

Since the 1960s, women in Quebec and in Canada have increasingly had better access to education and the job market. They have also made gains in autonomy, particularly with regard to conjugal status (whether or not to marry and choosing their partners) and protection (marriage contracts and right to divorce). This autonomy stems in part from gains in reproductive freedoms, with access to contraception and abortion services. The arrival of the birth control pill is considered one of the most significant scientific advances of the 20th century. It directly impacted the women's liberation movement, both in Quebec and around the world. The pill transformed the relationship between women and men, along with the family structure. Changes to the status of women were reflected in their fertility, particularly in Quebec; women today give birth to fewer children and have them later in life. In 2017, the average age of a mother in Quebec was 30.64.[4] This average advanced age for childbearing affects women's fertility, leading to an increase in the use of reproductive interventions.

Women are not the only ones to have gained access to rights; they paved the way for other social groups like children, the disabled, and those suffering from mental health issues. And it doesn't stop there. Today, more and more members of minority groups are demanding that their rights be recognized. A notable example is the prohibition of discrimination based on sexual orientation.

The evolution of the family

Since the 1960s, secularization in Quebec, access to health services, and improved status for women have brought profound changes to the typical Quebec family. Today, an increasing number of children are born out of wedlock, and the rate of blended families is growing. Reproduction is now viewed as a personal issue, whereas before, it was considered a social requirement (and still is in many societies), taking place within an established religious union. Children born outside this union were regarded as illegitimate. Reproduction was a social duty: it was essential for population replacement and, in certain environments, children contributed to the family workforce, promising succession as well as continuity. Families were larger, birthrates not as controlled.

The status of children

The status of children has therefore also evolved, as Gilles Houle and Roch Hurtubise have shown:

> From the moment the conversation addressed childhood or children, we began to have fewer of them: reflective childhood became a choice. There has clearly been a

change in our reproductive habits. In the past, young people—in love or not—married and started a family. The young wife would soon be pregnant, or, to use a popular expression, "in the family way." Today, young people in love marry—or not—and decide whether or not they want children: not right now, later on, or maybe never. In all cases, not very many.[5]

The child is no longer considered an active participant within the family unit, but rather an individual with rights who must be educated and encouraged to flourish. In the past, a child gave back to the family and participated in communal tasks with a view to one day taking over. Today, the family "invests" in the child. We have greatly advanced the concept of child as an extension of self rather than of bloodline, and this status is part of a social context that shapes people's desire both to have a child and to use all possible means to do so. We must recognize this status to better understand why people claim the "right" to a child, a new reality that has prompted Jacques Testart, the biologist behind the first test-tube baby in France, to argue that the quest for a baby at any cost is ultimately a quest for "reproduction of self" rather than "procreation."[6]

Medicine and reproductive health

Beyond oral contraception, developments in medical, pharmacological, and technological knowledge have contributed to a social evolution on which they also depend. Interventions during pregnancy and birth have multiplied.[7] Procedures such as genetic counselling, prenatal testing, and foetal interventions have become normalized.

While women have always been subject to a certain level of supervision throughout pregnancy, never have they been so closely monitored—in most cases acquiescing out of a concern for safety. And the smaller number of pregnancies today encourages women to more readily accept their medicalization.

Health data confirms that medical intervention results in improved outcomes for mothers and children, a finding that contributes to their normalization. Maternal deaths have almost disappeared in the upper classes of high-income countries, and have decreased elsewhere. Perinatal mortality has also declined. Complications during pregnancy and delivery are better controlled. But it is easy to forget that these advances are not solely a result of medical progress; they can be attributed to improved living conditions and women's access to education, which can account for the higher average age of first-time mothers. These new conditions are combined with overall advances in prevention and healthcare.

As a result of this progress, methods for controlling reproduction have become the norm, including more efficient family planning; medically assisted reproduction; tightly monitored pregnancies that involve intervention; delivery interventions with a 25 percent rate of C-section in Quebec in 2017.[8] Rates of in vitro fertilization are very high. Since the first successful attempt in

1978, effectiveness has improved and its use has become widespread. Today, the idea that fertilization can occur outside the body no longer raises eyebrows.

Initially, the use of a surrogate was seen as an extension of these interventions, a possible "solution" for couples facing fertility issues (e.g., for women born without a uterus). Like other technical advances in human reproduction, the practice has evolved against a backdrop of social change. Grounds for the procedure need no longer be physical, as in the above example, but can be social—for instance, in the case of homosexual couples. If these couples, whose legal unions are now recognized, wish to have genetic children, they can enlist the help of a woman they know or use an intermediary to recruit someone to carry their child(ren), for remuneration or not, depending on the regulatory context in which the transaction will take place.

Sometimes people justify a surrogate by arguing that adoption is difficult or lengthy. When parents desire a genetic link with their child, adoption ceases to be an option. According to anthropologist Françoise Héritier, the value placed on this genetic connection represents a major sociocultural shift in human reproduction. "Most of the problems we encounter come from the introduction of the notion of biological truth and, more profoundly, the notion of a genetic truth, when establishing descent."[9] Héritier believed that in our quest for a genetic truth, possibly leading to autonomous reproduction, there looms a "danger from which humans have always been shielded: a society that does not resort to otherness to create social bonding."[10]

A confluence of social and cultural conditions, as well as scientific developments, made surrogacy a way for people to have children. Sylvie Martin observes:

> The current climate of moral relativism and "situational ethics" suggests that it is individual desires, coupled with technical potentialities and their promised benefits, that legitimately dictate the course of developments in biotechnology according to the "technological imperative" of "if we can, we must."[11]

Evolving knowledge and discourse

We must also consider how discourse surrounding gender and motherhood has evolved. At the heart of this discourse lie certain feminist and gender theories whose messages have become increasingly popular and have undergone major developments. The rooting of the construction of this discourse and its influence on our relationships may seem far removed from the technification of reproduction, and more specifically from the use of surrogate mothers. But this is not the case.

Simone de Beauvoir's feminist writing has had an incomparable effect on women's progress towards greater autonomy. Yet it has also influenced the representation of motherhood, which became a feminine experience of confinement. The objective of de Beauvoir's claim that "one is not born, but rather becomes, a woman"[12] was to denounce oppressive social

Uncorrected Galleys

norms, but it also suggested that motherhood could present an obstacle to women's liberation.

Simone de Beauvoir called for women to step back from the experience of motherhood, the potential for which is inscribed in the female body. Her words, in the name of the emancipation of women, have contributed to devaluing motherhood. This vision of motherhood, as seen by a woman who was, on the other hand, a great feminist, gave women a new ultimatum: to achieve self-actualization, they would have to forego motherhood. The feminist movement's efforts to favour access to education and paid work, in a context without the conditions necessary for work/family balance, forced women to choose between the two, otherwise their living conditions became difficult, not to say impossible in all areas.[13]

The association between motherhood and confinement thus became an integral part of some feminist discourses in the second half of the last century, though they were not without their critics. Here is what I wrote twenty years ago in response to some young women's concerns who, expressing the wish to become mothers, were told their choice could run counter to their autonomy:

> It is confinement to the domestic sphere, not the associated human experiences, that has posed and may continue to pose a problem. Accepting the devaluation of motherhood negatively affects not only mothers, but all women. Demanding another status for motherhood

Uncorrected Galleys

does not imply that it is all women's destiny. It affirms that motherhood is an experience unique and essential to humanity.[14]

Today, this negative association leads us to believe that new reproductive technology can liberate women by helping them bypass the requirements of motherhood. Author Marcela Iacub, a self-proclaimed feminist who is well known in France for promoting medically assisted reproduction, writes in her book *L'empire du ventre, Pour une autre histoire de la maternité* [The Belly Empire: A different story of motherhood, trans.][15] that she is awaiting the arrival of the artificial uterus. She ignores the psychological and social elements of the bodily experience and essentializes what she calls the "intention of becoming a parent." By subscribing to technological solutions to fulfil this intention, she opposes feminist theories that define the physical experience of motherhood (conception, pregnancy, childbirth, breastfeeding) as human and not simply mechanical. Jean-Hugues Déchaux, professor of sociology at the Université Lumière-Lyon-II, writes that Iacub's position reduces the status of the body to a mere instrument. In fact, the body's experience is not only material but also symbolic and imaginary, these dimensions being shaped by the human group to whom one belongs. Déchaux also asserts that the biological and symbolic spheres are "closely related and sociologically difficult to isolate."[16] In short, a current within feminism advocates a disembodied approach

Uncorrected Galleys

to reproduction, denying its experiential and humanly rewarding nature.

It is also important to consider gender theory. Current use of the term "gender" does not fit with de Beauvoir's vision, which argued for lifting restrictions imposed on women because they were women, not denying their biological sex.[17] But this use also plays a role in how representations of motherhood have evolved, along with representations of the sexes and their complementary nature in reproduction.

Below is the definition of gender according to Statistics Canada. Note that it refers to one's "gender identity," or the cultural representation of how a person identifies based on sexual stereotypes.

> *Gender* refers to the gender that a person internally feels ('gender identity' along the gender spectrum) and/or the gender a person publicly expresses ('gender expression') in their daily life, including at work, while shopping or accessing other services, in their housing environment or in the broader community. A person's current gender may differ from the sex a person was assigned at birth (male or female) and may differ from what is indicated on their current legal documents. A person's gender may change over time.[18]

What does this have to do with surrogate mothers? It concerns the body. Gender identity is now considered independent of biological sex; people can identify as male or female regardless of their sex. This differs from the concept of gender used in feminist theory to refer to cultural roles associated with the sexes. Feminist literature, developed in the wake of work done by American historian Joan Scott, aimed to challenge inequalities between the sexes based on roles attributed to each.[19] Today, the concept of gender involves claiming a gender identity based on sexual stereotypes and not defining oneself by the sex as embodied (which doesn't necessarily correspond to the gender one wishes to identify as). This denies the psychological and social experience of reproduction rooted in a biologically sexed body. This new discourse rationalizes the view that pregnancy can be replaced by a technical procedure stripped of all human, psychological, and social dimensions. Such a definition suggests that women who bear children are interchangeable. Moreover, this argument disregards maternal-foetal exchanges in utero, which we will come back to later.

Anthropologist Jérôme Courduriès uses a similar discourse when writing of pregnancy and childbirth:

> We cannot entirely reject the hypothesis that the relative occultation of men, in available data concerning pregnancy by gestational carrier, may be the result of a specific gaze used by sociologists and anthropologists who, like their peers, are imbued with the idea that pregnancy and childbirth is primarily women's business.[20]

Pregnancy and childbirth, "primarily a woman's business," is an idea. By disembodying a nine-month experience followed by childbirth, in addition to the preceding physical experiences (such as menstruation and ovulation) exclusive to women, it is possible to conclude that pregnancy and childbirth is not an issue that concerns women in particular.

Here is an edifying intellectual exercise that reduces the human experience of motherhood to its physical condition ("gestation") and offers a representation of this experience that paves the way for the ultimate technification of human reproduction. Seen like this, mothers could essentially be replaced by machines. This perspective also likens sperm donation to ova donation, which is a more complex and riskier process requiring medical intervention.

Neoliberalism and globalization

Other elements, in addition to those mentioned above, come into play on a broader scale: the global economy. Neoliberalism, the free market rule, and the valorization of economic efficiency (defined in terms of the capital and gains of certain actors) put the individual first. As a result, there are fewer collective options that benefit the general population. In this context, reproduction is left to often poorly regulated markets where the rich take advantage of the poor for personal gain. There is increasing support for individual rights, and this widening scope is more often dictated by an essentially individualistic approach rather than by a humanistic perspective associated with respect for human dignity. The value placed on reproductive intermediaries is indicative of how significant the market economy has become in social life.[21] The moment reproduction entered the trade market, intermediaries appeared and began to make profits from it. Today, business is booming wherever gamete donation and the use of surrogate mothers is authorized.

Globalization opens borders and increases exchange between societies and cultures. Without tight regulation and a concern for the common good, neoliberalism fuels a rise in the resulting inequality. Surrogates frequently come from low-income countries, while the commissioning parents are from high-income countries. Added to which is the difficulty governments have legislating and applying the laws, which are easily circumvented by going elsewhere, where different rules apply. This is the case in Canada. The principle of extraterritorial jurisdiction of the Criminal Code only applies to certain cases, such as child sex tourism or human trafficking. This issue is central to the debate over surrogacy legalization. Since Quebec does not recognize a contract as valid, go to Ontario! Canada tolerates surrogacy without remuneration, but then you just have to go south of the border or... somewhere else.

Today's reality

While the incidence of surrogacy has increased considerably in recent years, it is difficult to assess to what extent. Information is patchy, especially in Canada, where researchers complain that statistics are either lacking or invalid. Legislation and jurisprudence differ

Uncorrected Galleys

between and even within countries, which is the case for Canada. This situation favours "fertility tourism to more permissive environments."[22] And the rules are constantly changing. It is impossible to get an accurate picture of the issue, especially since surrogacy is not regulated in certain areas and therefore lacks documentation.

Regulations surrounding surrogacy are in constant evolution. Some places are tightening rules while others, like some U.S. states, are becoming more permissive. Previously lax Asian countries are now imposing stricter controls, such as making surrogacy inaccessible to foreigners, which shifts the demand along with a progression of surrogacy to regions that are more permissive and less regulated. This mobility is reminiscent of profit-hungry multinationals that withdraw from countries where workers' organisations have mobilized and labour laws improve in favour of those with less worker protection.

At this point, it is important to recall the two types of surrogacy: the free, so-called altruistic model, and the commercial model. And as with anything divided into "types," many possible variations of each exist.

In the first case, the surrogate agrees to surrender, without remuneration, the child she has just birthed. Examples of this practice include women acting out of friendship or familial support, who receive nothing in exchange for the child. But in reality, this is rarely the case; "altruistic" arrangements can vary considerably.

Though a woman may not be explicitly remunerated, some agreements include provisions and compensation comparable to an income. And being "altruistic" does not mean there are no intermediaries. In Canada and elsewhere, commissioning parents may pay agencies to put them in contact with a surrogate. The hypocrisy is that these agencies exonerate themselves by claiming they do not remunerate surrogates, since doing so is illegal.

In the second case, which is the most common worldwide, surrogacy is commercial. A signed agreement between the future surrogate and the commissioning parent(s) includes remuneration for "services." These contracts contain different degrees of detail regarding the surrogate's habits (diet, etc.), behaviour (sexual relations, freedom of movement), and rights (termination of pregnancy, breach of contract, custody arrangements). Contracts also vary: certain American women may be treated and paid well, while the conditions of those from India, Nepal, or Thailand can be compared to those of slavery, considering the definition stated in article 1 of the United Nations' Slavery Convention: "Slavery is the status or condition of a person over whom any or all of the powers attaching to the right of ownership are exercised."[23]

When it comes to commercial practices, intermediaries act as a liaison between the commissioning parents and the surrogate, not only for recruitment and selection of features (which may involve purchasing ova from another woman), but also for the following stages. This may include supervising the mother and overseeing contact between the two parties; organizing prenatal care (with total control over the surrogates in certain regions); birth; and "delivering" the child to the commissioning parents.

Commercial surrogacy is well developed in some U.S. states and in many emerging or low-income countries because it is a lucrative industry. In these countries, limited access to the labour market or poor working conditions for women make a paid pregnancy very attractive.

In places where surrogacy is prohibited, advocates for its legalization tend to support defined regulations while maintaining a ban on the commercial practice. Yet "altruistic" surrogacy occupies a grey area when it comes to compensating the women. Will regulations be enough to dispel doubts? Probably not. Will legalization encourage other, more or less commercial, forms of the practice? Very likely. We can see it happening in Canada already, where unpaid surrogacy has been available for a number of years and companies serving as intermediaries are well established.

Moreover, using the court system is an effective mechanism for ensuring the transition from the "altruistic" form to the commercial one, as well as the transition from the prohibition of the practice to the acceptance of an "altruistic" form. French legal expert and regulation specialist Marie-Anne Frison-Roche describes this mechanism as a way to "dodge the power of the legislature by seducing the jurisdictional authority."[24] It works as follows: people are unable to get what they want in one place (i.e., in Quebec, where surrogacy is prohibited, or in Canada, where only unpaid surrogacy is legal) so they turn to other, more tolerant environments—like former President of the Treasury Board Scott Brison did.[25] Once they come back with the child, they turn to the courts, which operate on a case-by-case basis, to sanction their actions. This prompts surrogacy advocates to call for regulation by way of legalization, since judges are presented with *faits accomplis*.

Surrogacy and the law

From a legal standpoint, countries are situated along a continuum that ranges from a ban on surrogacy, to differing levels of regulation, to complete silence (i.e., total permissiveness). The global portrait is constantly evolving, making it difficult to get accurate, up-to-date information.

In 2018, the report submitted to the United Nations Human Rights Council gave an account of the situation, drawing on numerous references for support:

> National laws governing surrogacy vary across a spectrum from prohibitionist to permissive. This variation occurs across national boundaries and sometimes within national boundaries, as surrogacy is sometimes regulated primarily by local law (i.e., in Australia, Mexico, and the United States). The most prohibitionist jurisdictions,

such as France and Germany, ban all forms of surrogacy, including commercial and altruistic, and traditional and gestational. Most jurisdictions with laws governing surrogacy, including Australia, Greece, New Zealand, South Africa, and the United Kingdom, prohibit "commercial," "for-profit," or "compensated" surrogacy, while explicitly or implicitly permitting "altruistic" surrogacy. Only a small minority of States explicitly permit commercial surrogacy for both national and foreign intending parents, thereby choosing to become centres for both national and international commercial surrogacy. Cambodia, India, Nepal, and Thailand, and the Mexican State of Tabasco, are examples of States or jurisdictions which have served as centres for commercial international surrogacy arrangements but have recently taken steps to prohibit or limit such arrangements, generally in response to abusive practices. However, Georgia, the Russian Federation and Ukraine, and some states in the United States, have for a sustained period of time chosen to remain centres for international surrogacy arrangements.[26]

In the absence of legislation (such as in Belgium, a prominent example in Europe), decisions fall to the courts. Verdicts then rely on rulings within the context of family law.

On an international level, the situation is quite complex. If one country prohibits or sufficiently regulates surrogacy, commissioning parents will go elsewhere. The report submitted to the HRC notes that:

Countries that have changed course by prohibiting commercial surrogacy		
Country	Date ban went into effect	Regulations
Cambodia	2016	
India	2016	Altruistic surrogacy is accessible to Indian nationals who meet certain conditions: heterosexual couples who have been married for at least five years experiencing infertility, only allowed between close relatives, no payment beyond reimbursement.
State of Tabasco (Mexico)	2016	Altruistic surrogacy is accessible to heterosexual Mexican nationals.
Thailand	2015	Altruistic surrogacy is accessible to married heterosexual Thai nationals who meet certain conditions: a close relative or a woman between 20 and 40 who is already a mother.
Vietnam	2015	Altruistic and gestational surrogacy limited to certain conditions: couples must prove their infertility and register with a government agency, women can only be surrogates once, and monetary reimbursement is limited to medical bills.
Nepal	2015	
Countries where surrogacy is legal		
Country	Rules (or lack thereof)	
Kenya	No formal law; a few protective measures exist regarding birth certificates and consent of surrogate mothers upon adoption.	
Laos	Surrogacy practice is developing as a result of restrictions established in Cambodia.	
Malaysia	No current legislation; a fatwa was issued prohibiting the use of surrogates, leaving states free to abide by the injunction as they see fit.	
Nigeria	Criticized for its "baby factories,"* all surrogacy agencies have been shut down but the commercial practice is still authorized.	
Russia	In 2011, non-genetic surrogacy was legalized for married heterosexual couples or infertile women; surrogates are required to have had at least one child and may become legal parents upon the child's birth, despite any agreements formed with the intending parents. In Russia there is opposition to both altruistic and commercial surrogacy.	
Ukraine	Commercial surrogacy is limited to married heterosexual couples, but the commissioning parents are recognized as the child's legal parents and no adoption process is necessary.	

* "Nigeria police raid Lagos 'baby factory,'" *BBC News in Africa*, 30 September 2019, https://www.bbc.com/news/world-africa-49877287.

The cross-border patterns of international surrogacy arrangements are diverse. Commonly, intending parents from developed countries, including Australia, Canada, France, Germany, Israel, Italy, Norway, Spain, the United Kingdom of Great Britain and Northern Ireland, and the United States of America have engaged in commercial international surrogacy arrangements with surrogate mothers in developing countries, such as Cambodia, India, the Lao People's Democratic Republic, Nepal, and Thailand. However, California and other jurisdictions in the United States are centres for commercial international surrogacy arrangements, as are Georgia, the Russian Federation and Ukraine, creating a different set of cross-border relationships. In addition, intending parents from China frequently engage in commercial surrogacy in South-East Asia and the United States. All of these patterns pose human rights concerns.[27]

The Chinese example is particularly interesting. China's one-child policy was in effect from 1979 to 2015, and since it was eliminated an estimated 90 million women have been permitted to have a second child.[28] Since there remains a national preference for boys and since prenatal sex selection is banned, Chinese couples have begun turning to foreign clinics.[29]

In Europe, twenty of the twenty-eight member states oppose the practice of surrogacy. The exceptions are Belgium, the Netherlands, Poland, Slovakia, Romania, Ireland, the United Kingdom, and Portugal, where access to intervention differs.

In areas where surrogacy is currently prohibited, there are movements pushing for its legalization. The debate rages most notably in France, where one group firmly opposes legalization and another firmly advocates it. We will revisit the arguments themselves in further chapters; they are more or less universal. One side makes a case for human dignity, opposing the instrumentalization of women and commodification of children. The other side views surrogacy as proof of how families are evolving and an indication of social progress.

The American website Surrogacy360.org[30] provides up-to-date information on international surrogacy. This is useful since regulations are constantly changing. It includes a list of countries that have introduced legislation in response to abusive practices. Many of these countries were featured in news reports denouncing the treatment of surrogate mothers. As a result, some now ban commercial surrogacy while others have introduced stricter regulations.

The situation in the United States is more complicated. Surrogacy is regulated at the state level, resulting in a wide range of possibilities. Françoise Dekeuwer-Défossez, a professor of private law at the Université Lille-2, notes:

> The exemplary case is the United States: the lack of federal legislation concerning family law, together with the inherent jurisprudential nature of American law, leads to a collection of disparate and inconsistent decisions for

which only a shrewd interpreter would be able to find a common thread … other than a confrontation between the law of the market and the law of God…[31]

For its part, the website Creative Family Connections[32] offers an interactive map of the United States detailing commercial surrogacy laws by state. This pro-surrogacy service warns prospective parents that laws governing surrogacy vary, not only between states and even between counties within the same state, but also between how the law is written and how it is actually practiced in these areas. States are grouped into five categories, from those with the most permissive laws to those with the most restrictive laws. The vast majority fall under the former classification, with only three considered very restrictive—some of which do not recognize formal contracts between commissioning parents and surrogates. In practice, however, cases to establish parentage have been brought to court. It should be noted that the website uses the term "pre-birth order," which likens ordering a baby to making a purchase on Amazon.

As countries offering cheaper options begin to close their doors, commissioning parents are turning to Canada.[33] Economic factors now make Canada a competitive force to rival the United States, despite the wide availability south of the border. Surrogacy is cheaper in Canada, particularly when it comes to the health care bill.

Exploitation of needy women from poor
countries and negative fallouts

Surrogacy sparks much debate, even among groups
that agree with it in principle, since some practices
are condemned as outrageously dehumanizing, sometimes criminal. According to the report submitted to
the HRC in 2018:

> Abusive practices in the context of surrogacy are well
> documented. Examples include convicted sex offenders
> from Australia and Israel employing surrogate moth-
> ers from India and Thailand, a wealthy Japanese man
> employing 11 surrogate mothers, leading to the births of
> 16 infants in Thailand and India, the abandonment of a
> surrogacy-born infant with disability in Thailand, and the
> abandonment or sale of "excess" surrogate-born infants
> in twin births in India. Commercial surrogacy networks
> transfer surrogate mothers, sometimes while pregnant,
> across national borders in order to evade domestic laws;
> in one case, 15 Vietnamese women were found and freed
> by Thai authorities, leading to human trafficking charges
> in the context of a baby-farming scheme.[34]

In simpler terms, here is how far the evolution
of practices can take us when commissioning parents resort to cross-border surrogates: ova from white
women are valued on the international market and are
"donated" or sold to buyers, regardless of their origin.
Once acquired, they are fertilized in vitro with the
sperm of the commissioning parent(s). The resulting
embryos are implanted into a woman's uterus, regard-

less of her skin colour. Freezing embryos facilitates
the operations, as it allows them to be transported to
countries other than where the in vitro procedure took
place. Choosing where to carry out the pregnancy is
often dictated by its price tag and how easy it will be
to leave with the child. In short, the surrogacy process
depends on access to two humans: one woman for nine
months and an unborn child for whom proof of parentage is required.

India

India was once something of a grim laboratory for surrogacy. A thriving and lucrative commercial market
was quick to develop, making the country a top choice
for commissioning parents. In 2016, abusive practices
led authorities to ban access for foreigners, and a prohibition on all commercial surrogacy quickly followed.
In December 2018, India's lower house of Parliament
passed a law imposing strict conditions on surrogacy.
Today, a surrogate must be a close relative, and the practice is limited to childless Indian couples who have been
married for five years and have a doctor's note certify-
ing their infertility.[35]

Until that point, surrogates were cared for throughout their pregnancies and industry norms had guaran-
teed commissioning parents that pregnancies would
be safe. Studies documenting the surrogates' experience showed that many were paid beyond what would
have otherwise been accessible to them. But the prac-

tice was also plagued by abusive treatments of women
and a flagrant inequality in power relations based
on class. People began coming forward to denounce
the treatment of surrogates. The most famous critic
is probably Sheela Saravanan, a research associate
from India currently working in the Department of
Anthropology at Heidelberg University in Germany.
In 2018, she published *A Transnational Feminist View
of Surrogacy Biomarkets in India*,[36] a critical study of
the pre-2016 "surrogacy bazaar" that draws on her
ethnographic work with surrogate mothers, commissioning parents, and medical practitioners. In it she
reveals prices were set based on a woman's reproductive capacity, her caste, her religion, and the number
of children born along with the babies' weight and
sex. Saravanan exposes breaches in consent and medical ethics and calls attention to basic human rights
violations.

The situation in India has provided a more detailed
picture of the dangers and abusive practices linked to
surrogacy, and it has shed light on the complex nature
of women's experiences. While these women subordi-
nated their bodies to the project of strangers, they found
a kind of emancipation through an otherwise inaccessible income and, in some cases, a previously unknown
access to care. They also found the ability to give someone else a child very rewarding. Nevertheless, exploiting
these benefits cannot counterbalance the conclusion of
researchers like Sheela Saravanan who consider that as

a violation of fundamental human rights, and from a
child rights perspective, the practice must be banned
globally.

Uncorrected Galleys

Chapter 2

Women's Issues

Women are now invited to participate in human reproduction no longer as the main actresses, but as supporting, almost interchangeable ones. Their role is changing. What are the consequences of this shift?

Experiencing motherhood

French sociologist Martine Segalen describes the recent evolution of motherhood as follows:

> Although biotechnological advances in the 1970s and 1980s—such as the pill and medically assisted procreation—greatly benefited women, they are now turning against them, with a globalized market that is taking possession of their procreative faculties, transforming them into a contract service.[1]

To accept surrogacy as a practice means defining pregnancy and childbirth from a utilitarian perspective, as inconsequential biological events; any woman can carry any child, since all she is doing is "gestating."

This representation trivializes pregnancy and child-birth, rendering them anonymous experiences and stripping them of a relational quality. Moreover, it likens the process to a job.

This perspective contradicts a different vision of pregnancy and childbirth as a global and relational human experience affecting body, mind, and senses. These are experiences that mark a life. Why are they so meaningful? Because carrying a child engages a woman physically, psychologically, and socially over a number of months. Pregnancy is not an activity, but rather a state of being; the pregnant woman is doing more than just making something. Pregnancy has significant physical and psychosocial impacts on the woman and child,[2] and its complex nature invalidates any comparison to performing a job.

This vision positions the woman, engaged in reproducing another individual, as living a human experience and not as a baby-making machine. The difference between the two lies in the very essence of humanity: consciousness, along with an ability to form relationships. These cannot be separated from the act of reproduction.

Pregnant women are aware of the child project they carry within them, a project that has a beginning, then grows and develops until it takes shape in a new being. The experience is not trivial or unremarkable. It bears the stamp of humanity, including an awareness of otherness: the woman's body houses a life that will be different from her own. Once outside its mother's womb, the child is a person separate from mother and father.

Human destiny is also part of this plan in the consciousness of life's finiteness. Not only does pregnancy and childbirth pose risks for both the mother and the child,[3] but the woman also knows the life she creates will end one day, just as hers will.

Until recently, a child was conceived when two people—the mother and the father—had a sexual encounter that may have been furtive or part of a broader narrative involving a happy, unhappy, tragic, or trivial story. The pregnancy and the resulting child originated from a human connection, a relationship marking the experience.

When artificial insemination became available, this connection was no longer necessary. Conception could be anonymous. Then, a major milestone was reached with the use of in vitro techniques: fertilization of a woman's ovum with the sperm of a man, likely a perfect stranger, followed by embryo implantation into the uterus of a surrogate. This changes the entire experience. The woman has not conceived the child she is carrying and has no connection to the father. Reproduction without sexuality is now fragmented. A woman's body can be used without regard for her humanity.

The international process that has become the norm for surrogacy uses gametes from two people who do not know each other (and who often come from different backgrounds) and engages a surrogate who knows neither. Thinking that this method eliminates interactions in utero is a mistake. Beyond cellular exchanges, we now know a woman's prenatal experiences do affect a developing foetus.[4] Considering the ovum donor to be the child's sole maternal biological link disregards exchanges in utero.

Reproduction of this nature is divorced from the act of sex as well as the overall experience of motherhood. The woman is instrumental, and her experience during the months of pregnancy is not often followed by a relationship with that child.

Could we cut out the mother completely?

Surrogacy is the culmination of an evolution that has seen the woman's role in childbirth gradually diminished. It therefore transforms the relationship between men and women, at the heart of which has always been reproduction, as pointed out by Françoise Héritier:

> It is not only because women have the privilege of giving birth to children of both sexes that it is necessary to appropriate their fertility, share them amongst men, and constrain them to domestic tasks related to reproduction and group management, all the while devaluing these particular roles—furthermore assuring women's subjugation by keeping them ignorant—but rather for a similar, yet very different reason. It is because, in order to perpetuate himself, a man needs a woman's body. He cannot do it himself. And this inability seals the fate of women everywhere.[5]

With surrogacy, the role of mother, once active in conception and throughout pregnancy, becomes fragmented and depersonalized. When a woman is inseminated to carry a child she will ultimately surrender—and even more so if her role is limited to the months of pregnancy—her experience is depersonalized, her female potential is instrumentalized.[6]

Men still need women to reproduce, but now they are able to do so excluding any human encounter. On a symbolic level, science has allowed them to reproduce alone. With no need for a mother, the woman is but a necessary cog in the wheel; the procreator now takes centre stage. This fragmentation, ending the certainty that the mother is the one who gives birth, prompts a fundamental question: who is now the mother? The woman who provided the ovum? The woman who carried and birthed the child?

To understand this evolution, let us examine the next planned step: the use of an artificial uterus,[7] completely eliminating the mother from the equation. In this scenario, the woman's ova will be fertilized in a lab and the resulting embryo will be left to grow in a machine. Women's bodies will no longer be needed to bear children, the logical conclusion of a type of reproduction that began with in vitro fertilization.

When we remove the mother, a woman's contribution becomes the same as a man's: to supply the gametes. Her body is no longer the site of reproduction.

We aren't quite there yet, but access to surrogacy has already upset a balance in gender relations.

Using a woman to bear a child, only to more or less erase her from the child's life, can be viewed through the technological lens: *since we can, we should.* But shouldn't we question how surrogacy is rooted in social relations and therefore how it impacts the lived experience of the participants, along with society in general? Should we accept a technique on the basis of its feasibility? Some say yes, since science helps to make a wish or a will come true; they cannot (or do not want to) reproduce without medical intervention. But others like French anthropologist David Le Breton disagree.

> Procedures made possible through biotechnology require, among other things, collective deliberation, an examination of viewpoints and values, and political arbitration. Ethics is not a transmission belt of a medical practice that continues to dictate its conditions by the growth of its power over the living. The Law cannot amount to technical and scientific data records. What is feasible is not necessarily legitimate.[8]

I am among those who disagree, because I am convinced that by developing this system, we endanger the human quality of reproduction and undermine the very foundations of our humanity. Surrogacy raises determinant issues for women, as well as for gender relations as a whole.

Reproduction and social bonds

Surrogacy is inherently depersonalizing since it eliminates the relationship between mother and child. Surrogacy contracts contain clauses that are intended to prevent this relationship from forming; otherwise, surrendering the child might prove too difficult. Such conditions run counter to reproduction's human character. Commissioning parents must take measures to prevent the development of the usually taken for granted mother-child bond and which, under other circumstances, would be strongly encouraged by perinatal services. The idea is to substitute a bond with the commissioning parents. Separating a child from its mother can sometimes be necessary, for example in cases where she is unfit or other potentially harmful situations. But this is by no means the case if the separation is definitive and planned prior to conception.

A 2016 study published in *Nature Neurosciences*[9] casts doubt on a claim to a depersonalized pregnancy. The authors compared women who have been pregnant with those who have not and found that pregnancy causes long-lasting changes to a woman's brain. These changes predicted measures of postpartum maternal attachment, suggestive of an adaptive process serving the transition to motherhood. The study highlights the biology behind the mother-child bond, which runs counter to the vision of a pregnancy detached from the body. According to French philosopher Laura Lange:

Uncorrected Galleys

Based on the idea that pregnancy does not make a mother, surrogacy paints a portrait of a body that can be mastered whose experiences can be anticipated and controlled. […] If surrogacy reinforces a desire to master the body's lived experience, then what about the meaning of the primary relationship that is formed and played out with the other within the womb?[10]

We must be careful not to make too much of this phenomenon; the mother-child bond does not guarantee the quality of the ensuing relationship. Different circumstances may intervene and harmony in the relationship cannot be assured. Yet observing the way a mother's brain changes can attest to the complex nature of pregnancy and its relational aspects, reinforcing its status as a human experience that should not be trivialized.

The technification of childbirth and...of the rest

The progress of technical interventions in reproduction has come at a price—they challenge the human aspect of the pregnancy experience. Women have, by their adherence, participated in the gradual technification of childbirth because they have been convinced that more control means less associated risk. And they were right. But an imbalance arose once the superiority of technology over the natural process was assumed and prompted a movement to humanize birth care and recognize the midwifery practice. Women began to feel the rise in medical interventions during pregnancy and childbirth was dehumanizing their experience, and they wanted better.

This protest movement, which was particularly active in the late 1970s and 1980s, was part of a global one. The international women's health movement called for technology to play a supporting role as opposed to being used as a primary approach.[11] Women argued that pregnancy and childbirth were normal life events that offered enriching and rewarding experiences, and they wanted to welcome their children into the world in a gentler, more humane manner. In order to achieve this, they maintained, surveillance and surgical interventions should be the exception not the rule, and their use justified. Technology should serve humans, not stand in for them. Women also claimed recognition of their competence in maternity matters.

The demands to recognize the practice of midwifery are in line with this logic, as midwives accompany women throughout pregnancy and let them play the leading role during the actual delivery. The literature supported these demands, attesting to the richness and complexity of motherhood. It also documented how medicalized and technified reproductive experiences can be damaging to women's status and autonomy.[12]

The movement made gains in Quebec, which legalized the practice of midwifery in 1999; abandoned certain interventions (the enema); re-evaluated the use of others (the episiotomy); and redesigned hospitals to make them more inviting. Similar gains were made

Uncorrected Galleys

elsewhere in Canada.[13] Nevertheless, this movement has not been able to curb the heavy trend, especially with regard to C-sections: "After three decades of activism, many note that the initial goal of humanizing childbirth (centred on acknowledging the mother's authority and ability to bring her child into the world herself) has pivoted to one that 'humanizes' its medicalization,"[14] writes historian Andrée Rivard.

Support for the representation of obstetrical interventions as being superior to natural childbirth is determinant. Despite continued discourse focused on women's autonomy, which advocates respect and support rather than submission to medical control, it appears mothers themselves accept this representation. Underlying is their internalization of the representation of childbirth as a process fraught with risk, one that requires close supervision. Yet critics, including doctors, continue to challenge birthing practices, especially when it comes to high rates of C-sections.

The techno-medical model of childbirth has developed progressively. Today, some women can be under the care of a midwife and give birth without medical intervention in a birthing centre. However, the majority of women get an epidural (62.4 percent) and one quarter deliver by C-section (25 percent in Quebec, 28.8 percent in Canada as a whole).[15] This control affects the quality of the birthing experience, fragmenting the process through the use of technology and gradually subjugating women. A medical and scientific authority took over pregnancy and childbirth, and women's expertise has paid the price.

We are now able to manipulate gametes, take action to define the product of conception, fertilize an ovum outside of the body, and monitor and intervene throughout pregnancy and during delivery. But none of this interference would be possible without a level of consent from women—and a cultural context with shifting social, economic, and cultural conditions.

Surrogacy marks a step backwards from the objectives pursued by the movement to humanize birth care. In this new role, women are not only more passive but also considered accessory. Technology cements this status by using different women's potential in the process. As a result, women are definitively instrumentalized.

Little is said about the fundamental issue: how technology can transform the reproductive role of both sexes. And yet, it shows the extent of the threat of dehumanization. When women demanded action in the face of increasing medical intervention, the term "humanization" was not just a figure of speech. It meant that reducing a woman's active contribution to childbearing diminished its human character.

A case for autonomy

The fight for women's autonomy is a fundamental step towards gaining recognition as "people" deserving individual and collective rights. It is what drives the struggle for women's right to decide what is best for them, particularly when it comes to reproduction. It encompasses family planning rights (when to have children, how many, and with whom), abortion rights, and respect for their decisions throughout pregnancy and during delivery. Autonomy has often been described as a woman's right to make decisions about her body. Such a claim must be put into context: women's bodies have long been appropriated by men and by institutions. This appropriation, which has marked social relationships throughout history, can still be observed today in many societies in the form of forced marriages, prohibition of divorce, and a lack of access to contraception or abortion, among other things.

When it comes to the debate over surrogacy, advocates often wield the feminist argument that women are exercising their right to autonomy when they decide to lend or rent out their body for pregnancy. But the use of this argument can be questioned, since this interpretation of autonomy does not stem from recognizing women as people. Exercising one's autonomy means being able to reproduce in conditions that respect human rights—and women should be treated as humans, instead of engaging in a relationship where they are instrumentalized. A woman who agrees to become a surrogate, thereby putting herself at the disposal of the commissioning parents and carrying a child she will surrender to them, agrees to submit to a degree of control over herself for nine months. Indeed, pregnancy is a state and she is not *doing* something, she is *being* the means to satisfy a demand.

To participate in such a project, women also have to give up an image of their body and its components as a whole. Instead, they must view their uterus as a piece of themselves—one they can decide to lend or rent out. One hypothesis to explain this representation is the use of ultrasound technology. Now a mainstream prenatal technique, it may have contributed to how women see and accept a fragmented vision of their body. Ultrasounds externalize what is internal. They externalize the foetus, making visible what up to that point could only be felt by the pregnant woman. Along with this symbolic fragmentation, the visual image may also contribute to a theoretical construction of reproduction that depersonalizes the body, justifying its use with no thought to its experiential and relational dimensions.

It is possible to remove certain body parts or other products (blood, sperm, ova) and donate them to another person. The uterus, however, is most useful while it is still inside a woman's body. This representation transforms the womb into a space to lend or rent, ready to welcome an embryo. Melinda Cooper of the University of Sydney and Catherine Waldby of the Australian National University describe this process as follows: "The uterus is technically and legally isolated as a component that can be contractually ordered, detached from the selfhood of the surrogate and repositioned in a production chain at the behest of the clinic and commissioning couple."[16] But in order for the foetus to grow, the woman's entire body is solicited—a reality she is aware of. These two researchers describe this representation as being at the heart of the transactions in India they analyzed:

> In short, the surrogacy contract requires both parties to agree that the surrogates' parturient biology can be both (semi)-detached and instrumentalized, in order to be rendered as an exchangeable, quantifiable entity. In the words of one clinician, "I inform [the surrogate] that ... I only need her uterus.[17]

The representation of the body, along with women's reproductive potential and childbearing experiences, are at stake.

Some ways of doing things are downright commercial and heartless, and can even be equated with slavery. Other arrangements are intended to be more amicable, leaving some room for the mother's decisions and including her in the conversation. Still others are drawn up between friends or acquaintances. But while humane approaches do exist, this does not change the underlying issue of using women for their reproductive capacity. The uterus is seen as an empty space to be rented out for the duration of a pregnancy, giving rise to the term "womb for rent." The expression "third-party reproduction," often used by advocates of so-called altruistic surrogacy, supports this representation that requires a woman to achieve its objective. If artificial wombs existed, the woman would no longer be necessary.

In October 2018, the symposium "Pour le respect des femmes et des enfants, abolir la maternité de substitution" (*To respect women and children, stop surro-*

gacy now) was held in Paris as part of the launch of the International Coalition for the Abolition of Surrogate Motherhood (ICASM). Jennifer Lahl, President of The Center for Bioethics and Culture Network, gave a presentation on surrogacy contracts. The contracts she cited were all signed in California.[18] It is chilling to hear how much control some commissioning parents seek over their surrogate's life.

Some of the contracts include clauses relating to diet, exercise, living arrangements, travel, and other activities. The surrogate may be required to 1) avoid forming, or attempting to form, a relationship with the child—this goes for her partner too, where applicable; 2) give access to her medical file, waiving the right to confidentiality; and 3) have sexual relations only with her partner, who must be medically screened. In some contracts, the surrogate must agree to terminate the pregnancy at the discretion of the commissioning parents, with the exception of gender selection or reduction in cases of multiple foetuses.

One clause in particular illustrates the undeniable appropriation of the surrogate: in the event that the surrogate requires life support in her second or third trimester, she (and her partner, when applicable) agrees to be kept medically alive until the foetus is viable, taking into account the best interests and wellbeing of the child. It is the commissioning parents who decide how long to keep her on life support, based on professional recommendations and her family's desires.

Uncorrected Galleys

Such clauses might seem extreme, and indeed they are. Yet they highlight the underlying problem: a contract forces the surrogate into serving a purpose that is not her own. No matter how far she must go to change her lifestyle and meet the commissioning parents' expectations, she has given up her rights. And this is a flagrant violation of human dignity.

Dignity of the mother and child

This practice also calls into question the dignity of the unborn child, since it is recognized as the subject of an exchange. Justifying surrogacy by arguing that women are exercising their right to autonomy conceals the double issue at the core of the practice: first, how to respect the mother, who becomes instrumentalized and exploited for a space that is symbolically detached from her body; and second, how to respect the dignity of the child being born. Exercising one's right to autonomy must be placed within a human and relational context; the principle of dignity establishes certain guidelines. In the words of legal expert Bertrand Mathieu, human dignity "declares itself as an independent and external limit to exercising freedom."[19]

To talk about "giving" a child to someone implies a child can be owned, which is not the case. A woman does not own the child she gives birth to, no more than she was the property of her own parents at birth. She is nonetheless responsible for the child, given how dependent newborns are. She may entrust it to others if she is not in a position to carry out her duties as a mother. Yet this transfer of responsibility differs from the obligations of a surrogate, which involve a prior arrangement to cede the child. Despite this distinction, some still name this act as "a gift of" a child, as if a human life could be given away.

A job like any other?

Some feminists consider surrogates to be providing reproductive work for which they have every right to be paid. This approach derives from an attempt to gain recognition of domestic work, housekeeping tasks, caring for and raising children, and caring for dependents as responsibilities that are also social contributions. In other words, they are jobs that require compensation, possibly financial.

This logic is taken a step further when applied to surrogates, since it focuses on the woman's specific contribution: the child. Studies have drawn comparisons between surrogacy and other kinds of "women's work" on several levels—for example, the risks involved, the intimacy of the experience, and responsibility for the resulting product.[20] The main fault in this argument is that it uses the social contribution made by women (through domestic work and family care) to arrive at the claim that, if a woman is to be instrumentalized for someone else's gain, she ought to be paid for this. The surrogate is *being* pregnant, she is not *doing* something. This distinction justifies criticism that equates surrogacy with slavery rather than with performing a job.[21]

The surrogates' side

Why do women agree to become surrogates? Motivations can be grouped into three categories: to make a gift, to experience another pregnancy, or to earn money. These categories are not mutually exclusive, and a woman may have several motives.

To make a gift

Anthropologists have studied women who have acted as surrogates. Testimonies show that these women feel fulfilled; they believe they have contributed to a couple's happiness. The notion of a shared fertility stands out, as well as that of fairness. Some women consider fertility a question of justice, not nature, and that infertility is unfair. If the child is intended for a heterosexual couple, the surrogate's contribution can even be seen as evidence of women helping women. Women's studies professor Laura Harrison makes the following observation:

> The women-helping-women narrative is one in which surrogacy is framed as the ultimate levelling device between women, regardless of their socioeconomic status, race, nationality, or sexuality [...] The ideological work done through this discursive framing of surrogacy decommodifies the exchange of a child for money and appropriately genders both the surrogate (as the selfless,

altruistic giver of life) and the intended mother (who obtains the social rewards of motherhood).[22]

When women are motivated by giving and sharing, the act of relinquishing a child becomes, understandably, ennobled. Surrogates whose narratives echo this representation tell their story using language that indicates happiness. Their speech reflects this paradigm, and they describe a feeling of doing good.

These women do not feel exploited; they have an affirmative discourse that expresses their desire to accomplish something, and this something will give meaning, and more, to their lives. Delphine Lance, a doctoral student in anthropology at the School of Advanced Studies in the Social Sciences in Paris, describes the surrogates she met as part of research conducted in the United States and Ukraine:

> Like heroes who save lives, they highlight the fact that they create lives to make a positive impact on the lives of couples. The slogan *I make families, what's your superpower?* has become very popular on surrogacy forums.[23]

Some women report involving their spouse in the decision and informing their children, who approve; they describe a project that includes the whole family. Others are more private and undertake the pregnancy as a personal commitment. There is little documentation on children who are aware their mother is a surrogate. In interviews, several women have described how they made sure to include their children in the "gift"

Uncorrected Galleys

of the unborn child. This experience deserves further research, as we know little about the effects of surrogacy on families.

The decision to offer this "gift" may be a personal decision. But it is also the fruit of efforts by organizations to promote the practice. In Canada, this is evident with services such as Canadian Fertility Consulting whose website reads: Surrogacy is the most remarkable gift a woman can give.[24] The CFC touts the concept of a "surrogacy sisterhood" and even holds retreats for these women[25] as a way to share their experiences. Journalists and researchers who approve of surrogacy feature this type of personal account, describing these women as generous and acting out of compassion.[26] The stories are credible; the women talk about how their experience has made them grow. Other accounts, of disappointed women and bad experiences, are not unheard of. But the narrative of the "gift" dominates the conversation, ultimately representing an extension of the traditional discourse that positions women within a framework of generosity and self-sacrifice.

Experiencing pregnancy

Some women become surrogates because they enjoy being pregnant but do not want to have more children themselves. Says one, "I knew my family was complete, but I wanted to experience pregnancy again."[27] Other less explicit motivations vary, including atoning for an abortion or starting afresh. But for some, surrogacy is

really about the joy of reliving a pregnancy and enno-
bling this new experience by making it a "gift."

Earning income

Globally, commercial surrogacy dominates. Like ova
donation, it represents a source of income for many
women. And the worldwide demand for made-to-
order babies continues to grow with help from varying
legislation, lax enforcement of existing laws, and an
injection of foreign currency to certain markets. For
many women, surrogacy can be a way to survive, feed
their children, temporarily boost the family income for
a finite (sometimes rather long) period, purchase otherwise inaccessible goods, and more. As such, the prevailing discourse is centred on women's emancipation
and sense of agency. Advocates argue that surrogacy
empowers women and gives them access to economic
independence. And this is true. For some, surrogacy
offers a path out of poverty for a while and can even
be used as leverage within the family. Nevertheless,
these advantages cannot mask the exploitative power
of surrogacy, especially in underprivileged contexts; the
women are accorded little respect from intermediaries
who require their reproductive potential to become
richer. It doesn't take much imagination to find other
ways to promote economic independence and improve
the living conditions of these women.

   We shouldn't assume these women's intentions are
entirely commercial. The same discourse rooted in "gift-

ing" and "sharing" is often present in the testimonies of women who agree to become surrogates for remuneration. In other words, the experience does not seem to be a simple transaction where women are paid, even though, in some accounts, they talk about the child to be born with a great detachment. Intermediaries frame surrogacy as a way to help build a family, insinuating that the experience is more than just a source of income, thereby idealizing the use of their bodies.

One example in particular stands out. American military wives have adopted commercial surrogacy as a way to offer help and experience pregnancy while getting paid or, in some cases, just as a diversion while their partners are deployed. Sally Howard, an English journalist for *The Telegraph*, writes that the proportion of babies born to a surrogate whose spouse is in the military is around 20 percent, while these women represent less than 1 percent of all American women of childbearing age. Some of these women even carry more than one child. Howard profiles several of these women, including the wife of a Marine who became a surrogate after a chance meeting with a social worker employed by a local surrogacy agency. The woman describes their meeting as feeling "like fate": the money would allow her and her husband to pay off their debts and start a college fund for their children. Her husband was supportive, saying, "Your body's your body." She went on to give birth twice as a surrogate.[28]

No one can judge these women or their motives. We can, however, look critically at the (instrumentalized) nature of the pregnancies, their consequences for the child (who has become an object of exchange), and the intermediaries who make money from what resembles a sale. We can also argue that the collective social impacts are harmful to women and children—and that opposing the practice does not undermine a woman's right to autonomy.

What about consent?

Consent is at the heart of the surrogacy practice. Women must agree to and follow through with surrendering the child at birth. Though they are capable of consent, the nature of their commitment and the circumstances of the request make it difficult, if not impossible, to make an informed decision.

In Quebec, in Canada, and in most Western nations, an ethical approach to health care involves respecting a person's right to autonomy as well as the rules for obtaining informed consent. At no time must the person consenting to care be pressured into a decision. He or she must understand the consequences and be aware of the associated risks.

These criteria apply to cases of surrogacy, since the project affects not only the woman's life and health but also that of the unborn child. To exercise agency, these women must be equal actors alongside the commissioning parents or intermediaries. An imbalance of power will negatively impact the woman's ability to refuse or negotiate the terms of the agreement. But surrogates who come from a lower social class or are less fortunate than the commissioning parents engage in a *de facto* imbalance of power. Likewise, a lack of options (or considerably less lucrative options) for earning a living puts them in a position of vulnerability.

Informed consent also applies to relational and psychological conditions. A woman may be in a situation of vulnerability (for example, she feels the need to atone for an abortion) or of exacerbated sensitivity. If a natural phenomenon is taken for an expression of justice—a human construct—it may lead to exploitation. When a woman believes that infertility or an inability to reproduce is somehow unjust, she may feel it is her duty to restore that justice. Women should also be able to refuse an arrangement without fear of emotional blackmail or having their decision interpreted as self-serving or displaying a lack of empathy towards the eventual parents. Neither should their refusal imply a lack of responsibility when it means turning down a potential economic gain for their family. The discourse advocating "altruistic" or commercial surrogacy plays to these different situations, which calls into question a woman's right to autonomy and informed consent according to universally accepted ethical criteria.

Every pregnancy is unique. Any woman who has had more than one child knows this. Some pregnancies are smooth and easy, others more demanding. Beyond the physical experience, the psychological experience (a fundamentally human component) can vary from one pregnancy to another depending on conditions such as

Uncorrected Galleys

a woman's age, social context, interpersonal relationships, and more. A woman cannot predict with certainty how the pregnancy will unfold, how she will feel,
and how she will react when it comes time to surrender
the child. Obstetrician-gynaecologist Sylvie Epelboin[29]
calls this the "unpredictable nature of pregnancy" and
stresses that this unpredictability, along with the ran-
dom occurrence "of most complications involved in
pregnancy limits the decision-making autonomy of the
surrogate candidate."[30]

It is worth noting that debates surrounding regulations for surrogacy always address the issue of breaches
of contract. Can a woman change her mind? It is a necessary question when it involves giving up a child she
has just given birth to. A pregnancy lasts nine months;
how can we assume that nothing will change in this
time? The report submitted to the HRC in 2018 con-
cludes as follows:

> Any choice by the surrogate mother after the birth to
> legally and physically transfer the child to the intend-
> ing parent(s) must be a gratuitous act, based on her own
> post-birth intentions, rather than on any legal or con-
> tractual obligations.[31]

In Quebec, the Advisory Committee on family law
similarly defines one of its six key orientations to imple-
ment a framework on surrogacy:

> To ensure the protection of surrogates and to preserve
> the dignity of women who will act as surrogates, this
> legal framework will have to acknowledge the surrogate

mother's absolute right to terminate at any moment the parental project or not to pursue it following childbirth, regardless of the genetic origins that permitted conception of the child; in the same perspective, it will also have to recognize the right of the surrogate mother who agrees to surrender the child to reconsider her decision and to recover the child within a certain time frame following the birth.[32]

Are women aware of the health risks involved, such as the elevated rates of C-sections for surrogate pregnancies? Prior to signing the contract, are they informed of the increased risks for mothers as well as babies in births involving medical intervention?[33] This seems unlikely, especially when the surrogates come from poor countries. What about the commissioning parents, who come from more privileged backgrounds? One thing is clear: owners and operators of surrogacy clinics, along with health professionals, know the risks.

The debate should not be dismissed on the pretext that these women are autonomous, can choose, and are free to consent. Likewise, the debate must also focus on the specific nature of the request: months of pregnancy, including possible health risks and unplanned psychological changes. It is a reminder that surrogacy relies on the trivialization and dehumanization of pregnancy. This is a necessary condition to the claim that informed consent is possible when committing to a process with an unknown outcome—one that involves an individual's own human investment and a future human life.

Breastfeeding

Little is said about breastfeeding in cases of surrogacy. Yet even beyond the recognized health benefits to the mother and child,[34] breastfeeding can contribute to a positive mother-child bond.[35]

Like pregnancy and birth, breastfeeding is trivialized and drained of its relational nature. As anthropologist Jérôme Courduriès writes, "the nourishing relationship [...] is constitutive [...] particularly in the ideology of motherhood and of the mother-child bond."[36] He describes the breastfeeding experience as an ideological construction—a moment of physical closeness with the child when a mother offers her breast. This closeness does more than just "nourish"; it creates a bond through tone of voice, speech, touch, and so on. In his description of breastfeeding, Courduriès relies on the same argument that was applied to pregnancy; he writes as if to detach the uterus from the mother, reducing pregnancy to an essentially gestative process. In this view, breastfeeding is of value principally for its nutritional benefit, justifying the request of some commissioning parents:

> [...] without imposing it on their surrogate, they preferred, with her consent, that she nurse the child for the first few days of its life. The decision was prompted by current discourse surrounding the benefits of colostrum, the thick liquid rich in proteins and antibodies that is produced by the mammary glands during the final stages of pregnancy and first days after delivery.[37]

Uncorrected Galleys

Some surrogates agree to pump their milk and give it to the commissioning parents without seeing the child again. In cases of heterosexual couples, the woman may take hormones during the months leading up to the child's birth that allow her to breastfeed. Other parents turn to human milk banks, some supplied by donations, others trading it, sometimes even on an international market. The latter case risks exploiting impoverished women who depend on selling their milk for income, sometimes to the detriment of their own children, as has been observed in Cambodia.[38]

But above all, breastfeeding helps create the mother-child bond. In the logic of using surrogate mothers—not real mothers, a legal fiction, need we repeat—it must be avoided. Not only the commissioning parents but the surrogate mothers themselves participate in preventing a mother-child attachment. Delphine Lance details her observations of mothers in Ukraine and the United States:

> Curiously, if discussions surrounding surrogacy address the issue of gestational, genetic, and/or intentional motherhood, they leave little room for breastfeeding as fundamental to maternity. Yet for many of my participants, it is considered a line that "shouldn't be crossed." Some women have said they categorically refused to nurse the child. "Pumping is okay, but not breastfeeding," explains Natalia (surrogate one time, Ukraine). The skin-to-skin contact is perceived as "too intimate"; the problem is not the milk itself but the physicality of the process. Katerina (surrogate one time, Ukraine) told me, "I didn't

want to, it was too hard… I wouldn't have been able to let him go."[39]

And again:

For many women, nursing a child cannot be compared to gestating it. Sustaining a child by blood does not confer the status of mother; sustaining it by one's milk, however, makes a mother of the surrogate […] The combination of physical contact and giving milk render breastfeeding unimaginable for some women.[40]

Without a doubt, breastfeeding illustrates the affective nature of motherhood.

Uncorrected Galleys

Uncorrected Galleys

Chapter 3

The Child at the Heart of Surrogacy

We seem to forget that at the heart of surrogacy lies the child, its *raison d'être*. All energy is focused on the period before the child's arrival and subsequent appropriation, and this lack of concern cements its status as an object of exchange. The child's wellbeing, future, and all other considerations are practically absent from the discussion, which instead centres on its status with respect to the commissioning parents.[1] A collective concern for the child suddenly arises when it comes time to determine parentage if cross-national borders are involved. In Quebec, the child's "best interests" have been invoked on more than one occasion to grant commissioning parents their title.[2] But this argument only applies once the surrogate has surrendered the child. Why not challenge it when the contract is being drawn up? A 2017 French research mission noted:

> In cases of adoption, the question of a child's best interests is addressed before its possible adoption: the child, already born, is in need of a permanent adoptive family;

Uncorrected Galleys

in cases of surrogacy, the question of a child's best interests is addressed after gestation has already occurred. In other words, adoption is an institution founded on the child's best interests while surrogacy is a practice rooted in the interests of the initiators.[3]

As a society, we must be concerned with the life offered to these children after birth. They should be provided with conditions for positive development, with stability, and with opportunities to prepare for a bright future. Yet these conditions can vary greatly depending on the child's environment and on circumstances surrounding the birth.

Assisted reproduction: stability or separation?

Before the development of the scientific, technical, and medical knowledge that made the interventions surrounding the birth of humans more complex, nature had the final word when it came to procreation.

Anthropological studies show that natural reproduction has always been regulated in order to establish systems of kinship and descent. Some argue that engaging a surrogate mother is nothing new, and that there is no "right" way to reproduce. The observation that there has already been and still is circulation of children in so-called traditional societies could legitimize a child's transfer following a contractual agreement, in societies based on the rule of law. This logic seeks to establish a link with past procreative practices in order to make new practices acceptable.

Of course, this raises questions. The different forms of child circulation observed in traditional societies are rooted in specific cultural practices, and the wellbeing of the children must be considered in terms of the social and cultural context into which they were born and not in the absolute.

A child who is born into an environment where education is a collective responsibility does not grow up with the same reality or under the same conditions as a child born in the 21st century as part of a contractual arrangement. A child entrusted to infertile parents living in a traditional society cannot be compared to a child born following an agreement with a surrogate mother who surrenders it, nor to a child bought from a company, dealing with surrogate mothers in California or Asia.

Based on what we know, we can draw parallels with how some societies may once have designated guardians for their children. But the similarities end there. Never before have we relied on a notion of genetic truth (previously an impossibility), ova donation, or the use of another woman's body to carry a child.

Understanding our origins

A child does not ask to be born. But once born, it often asks where it came from. In the case of surrogacy, a birth mother must transfer the child to its commissioning parents. The woman who gave the child life—

though not her genes, in many cases—is effectively abandoning it. This is a reality that a child will likely try to understand even after explanations are offered, and will need to justify this abandonment in order to feel respected.

The relational aspect

We should question the ethics of a medical practice that prevents a child from developing a relationship with his or her birth mother. Isn't there a risk of maleficence? The biggest thing the child risks losing in cases of surrogacy is the relational aspect. The transfer from surrogate to commissioning parents calls into question the mother-child bond. That issue challenges us. Beyond the reasons motivating the surrogate's decision to relinquish the child and beyond the experience of the pregnancy, it is the human element of the birthing process, expressed by the mother-child bond, that the child has been robbed of.

The mother-child bond is not some psychologist's invention; it is a well-documented process, backed by popular and scientific observations. There is both a physical and psychological connection that develops while the foetus grows in the mother's womb. We have already explored the complexity of pregnancy and childbirth from a woman's perspective and its meaning as a human experience. Let us now turn our attention to the child.

We know that exchanges take place between a pregnant woman and the foetus growing in her womb. We also know that the foetus is sensitive to the experiences of the mother's body. Finally, writes obstetrician/gynaecologist Sylvie Epelboin, we know that at the time of birth, the child bears the traces of the woman who gave it life:

> The mother-child bond established during pregnancy [...] can no longer be denied. Whatever is believed about this bond, it is nonetheless difficult to imagine how, even prior to conception, we could schedule its rupture. Pregnancy is a time of hormonal and nutritional exchanges, maintained by the child's movements in the womb, ultrasound imaging, the time essential to the birth process. It seems inconceivable to disregard the affective aspects of key moments in pregnancy without consequences for the mother or child.[4]

To believe a child is not affected when removed from or abandoned by its mother, we must ignore the scientific evidence: not only that exchanges in utero exist, but also that being in the arms of the birth mother prolongs an experience which began during pregnancy. Without essentializing its impact on a child's stability, we can recognize that this experience is beneficial. Feeling the safety of its mother's arms significantly contributes to a child's wellbeing. All children should begin life with such equal chances. As French psychoanalysts Myriam Szejer and Jean-Pierre Winter write:

For children, being separated from their gestator at birth represents a radical break with what they have known. Their postnatal perceptions are completely disconnected from perceptions memorized while in their mother's womb: her voice, the sounds of her body and possibly the voice of the surrogate's partner if he spoke near her stomach throughout the pregnancy, and the family atmosphere. Everything that gives a newborn his bearing in the first moments of life and provides the basis for his primordial narcissism is deliberately confiscated from him.[5]

These words echo the sentiments of a surrogate mother whose experiences were the subject of a U.S. documentary.[6] In it, she claims to have noticed a difference in the baby's reaction to her and her partner's voices compared to the voice of the adoptive father, reacting only to the first two.

Planning the separation

This planned impediment to the development of the mother-child bond, in order to satisfy one's desire to have a child, is probably the most objectionable part of surrogacy. Commissioning parents want to avoid an attachment with the mother, which is why she may not even see the child. This purposeful separation prevents a relationship from pursuing between the woman and the child she carried and bore. Sylvie Epelboin asks:

How can one organize and condone the disruption that it would be for a child to see its own pregnant mother give (up)[7] her baby, despite all explanations? At what price, and for what benefit, can one ask a child to share its mother's generosity?[8]

Commissioning parents give children a host of "explanations" to justify the mother's absence, which must prevail over the mother-child bond. These include their desire to have a baby and/or raise a child with whom there is a biological link; the investment put into planning and waiting for the birth; the fact that other children aren't raised by their birth mothers and do not grow up traumatized; and how, in some societies, child circulation is considered normal and the practice of giving children to infertile couples is accepted by the community. But can these explanations ever really satisfy a child and obscure the will, present before birth, to take the child from its mother and, in many cases, sever all ties to this woman—or go so far as to conceal her identity? According to psychoanalysts: Myriam Szejer and Jean-Pierre Winter

> In cases of surrogacy, the only connection between pre- and post-birth are the words about one's history that will give meaning to one's life. While it is important to tell a child his story, close attention must be paid to the words used: one cannot predict how this particular child will be impacted by the truth of its history. Moreover, the surrogacy story is not limited to the lore of families themselves. It is also part of a larger story told about society.[9]

The now widespread option of using two women can ease the process of erasing the mother. As part of her work with gay couples, Martine Gross writes:

It is presumed the gestational mother could suffer from the separation if she carried a child that was genetically hers. This belief goes hand in hand with the idea that a child could feel its birth story as abandonment rather than a gift. In this context, the use of an oocyte donor helps allay concern that a "full" mother (who is both surrogate mother and genetic mother) would play too large a role in the child's story.[10]

Many of the fathers who participated in Gross's studies had chosen and insisted on maintaining a relationship with the mother, although this was not always easy:

> "So we wouldn't be ashamed of what we did" is one motivation linked to the social disapproval surrounding surrogacy, when it is associated with the commodification of reproduction and women's bodies. Maintaining relationships allows surrogacy to be framed as a kinship practice, not as a business transaction.[11]

The story of a child's birth, later recounted to him or her, is therefore a key element in the construction of the relationship of kinship and the possibility for the child to find meaning in his or her situation. Whatever the circumstances, planning the separation of a child from its mother remains a risk factor that calls for justification.

The child's origins

Any discourse designed to minimize the impact of abandonment must ultimately address a fundamental human question: where do I come from? In some cases, the child knows who its mother is and may even remain in contact with her. But most often, she disappears. In more and more cases, the child also has a "genetic" mother (the woman who supplied the ovum) that he or she knows nothing about. In Germany, ovum donation is prohibited in the name of the indivisibility of the mother. The basis for this decision is that it is in the child's interest to have only one mother and to avoid depriving the child, born from such a donation, of the links to its maternal genetic lineage.[12] Thus, proponents of so-called altruistic surrogacy, focusing on this sole issue, argue that settling this question of anonymity settles everything.

The surrogate mother's anonymity

There are few studies on children born to surrogates and not enough time has passed to properly assess the risks involved and long-term effects on the children.[13] However, we do have access to up-to-date information on the physical health of the surrogate mothers and newborns (addressed further on). We also have a great deal of information concerning the experience of children who were adopted or placed in institutions and their search for their biological parents—particularly their mothers. In light of this knowledge, it seems critical to prohibit anonymity, whether we are talking about children given up for adoption, born to surrogate mothers, or born of ovum or sperm donation. Besides, more and more circles are recognizing that every child should be

Uncorrected Galleys

able to know where he or she comes from. In Quebec, the Act to amend the Civil Code and other legislative provisions concerning adoption and the disclosure of information was adopted in 2017 following years of pressure from various movements. It relaxed confidentiality regulations that had been exercised up to that point during adoptions. We cannot compare the experiences of adoptees in Quebec born to single mothers or orphaned at an early age with those of children born to surrogate mothers, but we can draw parallels when it comes to the search for identity.

There is still much debate surrounding anonymity in cases of ovum and sperm donation and surrogacy. For many, opposition to these practices stems more from their anonymous nature than from the practices themselves.

Given—or abandoned?

As well as wanting to discover their identity, children who are given away or adopted might also want to know more about why their birth mothers left them or what they may have been feeling at the time. Elisapie Isaac, an artist from Salluit in Nunavik who was adopted at birth, revealed that fact during a fall 2018 interview to promote her new album and single, "Una," written for her biological mother whose identity she had always known. Isaac noted that after giving birth to her second child, she wanted to explore what her own mother had been feeling at the time of her birth.[14]

In the song, I tried to picture myself as a newborn. That isn't really done in my culture, you have to live in the moment. But I've always been in search of the truth, and it kept coming back to haunt me. Like a dizzy spell that never goes away.[15]

Children's rights

We should note article 7, paragraph 1 of the United Nations Convention on the Rights of the Child, the international reference on children's rights: the child shall have, "as far as possible, the right to know and be cared for by his or her parents."[16]

The exact meaning of "as far as possible" is open to debate. However, it is quite plausible (taking into account the provisions included in other paragraphs) that the obstacles made respecting this right difficult or even impossible. Furthermore, this article was not about adults making plans to become parents. Since surrogacy is a planned activity, it seems fair to question this impossibility given the context.

Let's take another look at the report submitted in 2018 to the Human Rights Council, which presents a thematic study on surrogacy and the sale of children. It was initiated to address concerns that, in some circumstances, surrogacy may be likened to the sale of children. This concept is defined in the Optional Protocol to the Convention on the Rights of the Child on the sale of children, child prostitution, and child pornography as follows:

[…] any act or transaction whereby a child is transferred by any person or group of persons to another for remuneration or any other consideration.[17]

The underlying principle is that:

[…] the sale of children is a serious harm and human rights violation in and of itself, without having to prove any other rights violation under the Convention such as sexual or labour exploitation.[18 and 19]

The study submitted to the Human Rights Council covers different situations: "both international and national surrogacy, traditional and gestational surrogacy, and commercial and altruistic surrogacy." It is based on what has been done on adoption and implies that when it comes to surrogacy, it is in a sense back to square one.

The international community cannot relinquish gains made in the development of child rights norms and standards, including those developed in the context of adoption. […] the international community has insisted that the best interests of the child be the "paramount consideration" in regard to adoption, created standards requiring strict regulation of the financial aspects of intercountry adoption, sought to protect vulnerable birth families, and denied that prospective adoptive parents have a right to a child.[20]

The report submitted to HRC describes the different conditions under which relinquishing a child to its commissioning parents can be likened to selling a child.

In this context, the report affirms, the right to the child does not exist:

> A child is not a good or service that the State can guarantee or provide, but rather a rights-bearing human being. Hence, providing a "right to a child" would be a fundamental denial of the equal human rights of the child. The "right to a child" approach must be resisted vigorously, for it undermines the fundamental premise of children as persons with human rights.[21]

This alleged "right to a child" is used in certain cases to demand access to medically assisted reproduction. This issue is addressed in chapter 4.

When a child does not meet expectations

Surrogacy arises out of a desire for a child, with contracts establishing rules in order to fulfil this desire. The surrogate must agree to certain conditions to ensure the pregnancy goes well and the baby is healthy. This concern for a healthy child is reflected in the control exercised over the surrogate for nine months, as stipulated in the contract. Conditions vary depending on the context; some relationships are built on trust, and some come with strict rules (as we saw in chapter 2).

However, nothing can guarantee the child will be perfect or as imagined—and no contract clauses can guarantee the child will be received with open arms upon birth regardless of his or her characteristics. So what happens when the child does not meet expectations?

This was the case[22] for one Australian couple who conceived twins via a surrogate in Thailand. One of the children was born with Down syndrome, and the parents decided to bring home only the unaffected twin. This story drew worldwide attention to surrogacy practices. Other controversial stories of a similar nature have since made headlines.

Advocates of surrogacy can easily downplay this kind of event that draws media attention by arguing such stories are extremely rare or that the commissioning parents in question are not representative of all people who use a surrogate. Both arguments are no doubt true. And yet, these cases prove that the practice itself can be compared to purchasing an item that may be refused on the grounds the product did not match the order. This is not what natural parents of disabled children would do. In fact, it is the relationship to the expected child that appears in a rather crude light in these "incidents"; this relationship is dehumanized.

The situation can be further complicated if, during the pregnancy, it is revealed the child will be born with a disability. In these cases, everything depends on the contract and the termination clause. All this brings to light the seeds of eugenics contained in medically assisted reproduction insofar as it makes possible to select a child's characteristics or terminate a pregnancy on the same basis. Let's not forget that choosing an ovum donor from a catalogue constitutes a form of gene selection, which is the foundation of eugenics. And earlier we discussed using donor ova from a white woman but paying no mind to the skin colour of the surrogate.

Advocates of surrogacy generally paint a positive picture of the commissioning parents' ability to provide a good future for the child. Since the practice is often costly, it is easy to presume they are capable of offering material comfort and access to a good education. But who is this discourse aimed at? Is it to convince one-self—and the different actors involved—that the modus operandi is justified, considering what will be offered to the child? Can such a narrative gloss over the fact that surrogacy creates a gap in a child's history it will have to fill?

The interaction of the commissioning parents with the intermediaries or with the mothers usually makes it possible to avoid addressing the legitimacy of a birth that is ultimately far from ideal for the child. Indeed, like intermediaries, surrogates who adopt a gift-centred discourse that focuses on a family project obscure the risks incurred by the child whose existence will be based on a transaction. We can imagine, moreover, that these women are not in a situation that allows them to worry about the future of the unborn child. Take, for example, an Indian mother who uses surrogacy to lift her family from poverty. Why should she be concerned about the future of the child she will relinquish to parents who are much richer and come from an environment where access to education and living conditions is easy?

Uncorrected Galleys

Do not do unto others what you do not want done unto you

This ethical principle observed in most cultures (not only Judeo-Christian traditions) often comes to mind when I think about children born to surrogate mothers. What could the commissioning parents have thought? Some may not have known their own mother, others may have had difficult relationships with theirs, and still others likely had a loving mother. This range of experiences is presumably represented among couples considering surrogacy.

Regardless of the relationship we have with our own mother now, as an adult, can we imagine ourselves as the subject of a contract with a give (away) clause? As Elisapie Isaac puts it, "I tried to picture myself as a newborn." This is not done in her culture, she adds, reminding us that social practices surrounding reproduction are strongly rooted in culture.

How many commissioning parents ignore or downplay the impact surrogacy will have on the child? It is human nature to wonder about our origins; all children do at some point in their lives. Haven't these parents gone through similar experiences in their own personal development? And if so, how can they feel comfortable with their decision? If they can imagine being the product of a signed agreement with a woman—in some cases a poor woman on the other side of the world—, how many can believe this would pose no problem, or at least one with an easy solution?

Proponents of so-called altruistic surrogacy refuse to compare their behaviour to commercial practices requiring an investment, practices that often exploit underprivileged women. Yet despite all the possible complicity between commissioning parents and so-called altruistic surrogates, the question remains unanswered for the child whose fate may not be an enviable one. An adult's desire for a child cannot hide the fact that surrogacy represents a transaction with a woman who will likely not be there to answer future questions the child may have. The child will probably want to know why its mother, at the request of other adults, planned to bring it into the world only to surrender it.

All surrogacy advocates, whether theoreticians, intermediaries, stakeholders, or parents involved, downplay the risks for the child who may search for his or her origins and search for meaning in a life made possible by a contract. The narrative woven around a desire is determinative; it implies that desire justifies using any means possible to obtain a child. Can this desire overshadow a concern for the child's wellbeing when it comes to the construction of identity? A promise to love, care for, and educate the child to the best of one's ability cannot erase the fact that the relationship was founded on the rupture of another: that of mother-child. It is also founded on an arrangement or contract not driven by the child's wellbeing, but by satisfying a will to have a child.

Some couples believe the child will understand it was desired more than anything else, and that this desire will be sufficient for its stability. But this perspective goes back to the couple and to their desire to justify a practice that eliminates another human relationship, the very first one: the relationship between mother and child.

Throughout the process of surrogacy, the child is largely forgotten. He or she is objectified and transformed into something we hope to "have." The report submitted to the Human Rights Council, to which we have referred extensively, confirms this concern by stating that there is a proven risk of exchange not unlike the sale of children, and that the use of a surrogate mother is part of a relationship that challenges human dignity.

The same report presents the position of the American Bar Association, which makes it possible to grasp the commercial nature and lack of concern for the human dignity of surrogacy transactions in several countries. The Association considers that commissioning a child for money constitutes a market, and that the market-based mechanisms have so far proven efficient. It recommends that any international instrument on surrogacy ignore human rights concerns, and it rejects regulation within the surrogacy industry.[23] The position of this conservative association is founded on a practice whose components lead to significant wrongdoings.

The lessons to be learned here do not concern the wrongs of those who promote trade and the market at all costs, but instead the nature of surrogacy itself, a practice that allows this to happen. We must not forget that the transaction between adults renders the child a commodity. Advocates of altruistic surrogacy cannot ignore this reality or hide the fact that it develops within commercial societies. The moment a society allows children to become the subject of a transaction, it allows their trade to operate within the greater economy, whether for money or not. The negative effects are only the consequences of what was accepted when consent was given to such a social practice.

Where is the child in all this? In the words of anthropologist David Le Breton, "The child, in this process, is the invisible hostage of decisions that will affect its entire existence."[24] Children did not ask to be born under these conditions, and efforts over the last fifty years to protect their human dignity must be renewed. It seems that all the work done in cases of adoption must start afresh.

Uncorrected Galleys

Uncorrected Galleys

Chapter 4

Wanting a Child
versus Human Dignity

When it comes to surrogacy, an arrangement between supposedly consenting adults, demand drives supply. Increasingly, this supply is organized by intermediaries. The arrangement can be in the form of a so-called altruistic agreement or a for-profit contract.

Advocates of so-called altruistic surrogacy argue that the profit-based contract is the problem: the practice can exploit women and children and put them at risk of inhuman treatment (e.g., when these children are rejected). While it may seem surprising, this is not the real problem, although it does increase the risk of abuses. The real issue is the contractual nature of a planned birth that enables the exchange of a child. Under certain conditions, this exchange can be likened to the sale of children.[1]

The very idea that a child can be brought into the world to fulfil a contract is disheartening, even before money, compensation, or remuneration is involved. And rightly so, since it challenges the notion that no human being—in this case a child—can be subject to trade. This is a key argument offered by Marie-Anne Frison-Roche, a French expert specializing in regulatory law, who opposes surrogacy. In recent years, she has written extensively on the issue[2] and participated in discussions across various forums opposing the regulation of an exchange that instrumentalizes women and commodifies children. American law professor Adeline A. Allen holds a similar position. In a 2018 text published by the *Harvard Journal of Law and Public Policy*, she argues that a contract is not an appropriate means of establishing a relationship that involves questions of "identity, origin, lineage, belongingness, loving, and longing."

When freedom of contract is applied to surrogacy contracts such that the parties' consent and intent govern, "[b]irth becomes the subject of negotiation, and motherhood is exchanged in the market." When birth mothers and children are thought of as raw material, they are reduced from whole beings to commodities. This coarsens us and dehumanizes us.[3]

Both legal experts oppose efforts to regulate surrogacy, since it is clearly problematic as a contractual agreement committing, on the one hand, nine months of a woman's life and, on the other hand, the existence of a child.

The issue of a contract is unavoidable, despite efforts to dress it up using other words. A contract does not necessarily involve money; it refers more generally to a commitment between two parties. Recognizing the legality of a contract in which a woman cedes her child after nine months of pregnancy, even when it does not involve compensation, renders the dehumanization of mother and child socially acceptable. Allen argues that surrogacy reduces the mother and child to commodities, even when the transaction is done with the best intentions and under the best circumstances. The harm that results is inherent to the practice, and no amount of regulation can change this fact.[4]

Although attempts to amend article 541 of the Quebec Civil Code stem from a desire to protect the child, they are nonetheless misguided. All types of surrogacy are declared to be null in Quebec, yet advocates want lawmakers to recognize such contracts as valid under certain conditions. In truth, nothing can humanize people who have been dehumanized by being made the subject of a contract. Proponents of surrogacy wield the "desire for a child" argument, which holds that their desire should justify the use of a contract. Let's examine this argument more closely.

Wanting a child

Procreation is essential to the perpetuation of life and the survival of the human species. The desire to become a parent and to have children touches on several dimensions including human relationships, affection, love, and the future. But why does this desire sometimes seem to be confused with a desire to reproduce at all costs (even if it requires a contract)?

The will to have descendants, even if it involves taking radical measures, is nothing new. History is full of stories of men appropriating and abusing women, in a context where social rules urged procreation, so they could produce an heir and pass on power, rights, and property.

What is surprising is that not much has changed, despite collective efforts over the past fifty years in societies around the world to promote the rights of women and children, who are so often treated without regard to their humanity. In fact, significant gains have been made on this score. So why is there a growing cry for surrogacy to be legitimized, when the practice continues to appropriate women's reproductive potential and routinely overlooks the child?

A wish to procreate has now become an unbridled desire for a child. This can be explained by a shift in values among societies that have made significant advances in biomedicine and reproductive techniques, coupled with a rise in individualism. Let us examine how the evolution of medical knowledge and technical skills has combined with the rise of individualism to foster a desire for a child that has become an irrepressible need to reproduce.

The children of biomedicine

Medicine has long been interested in fertility issues and their causes, and this interest has driven advancements in the field. There has been rapid progress made, and within a short time, in the collective imagination, fertility problems have become something that can be fixed. Where it was previously impossible, some men and women have become the parents they hoped to be.

Demand for medical intervention and industry response go hand in hand. As patients push for solutions, research seeks them out. The more we find, the more we intervene. And we are constantly testing the limits.

If using these techniques can produce these long desired and long awaited children, it also raises the dreaded question of parentage: who are the parents of children born of biomedicine?[5]

Anthropologist and ethnologist Françoise Héritier noted that in today's society, wanting a child is rather self-centred; in traditional societies, it was considered a social duty:

> [...] it [the child] is not intended as object of pure desire and appropriation, as consumer good and emotional investment for the couple or individual, even if it represents economic capital and, as has been noted, life insurance. It seems to be about a desire for bloodline and a desire to accomplish, rather than a desire for a child, along with a need to fulfil a duty towards self and the community rather than laying claim to one's right to own.[6]

Uncorrected Galleys

No one misses the days when, in our culture and many others, infertility earned a type of social condemnation. To be a woman, you had to be a mother. Once married, a woman had to get on with having children. At the time, infertility was incorrectly believed to be a woman's problem; men were rarely thought to be sterile. This era was tough on women, but also on childless couples—a reality that still exists in certain circles where couples are stigmatized for not having children.

Advancements in science and technology have led to a new imperative targeting mainly women: a duty to use all available means to procreate. This injunction applies not only to those who live in societies, such as ours, where women are free to choose or reject motherhood, but also to those who live in environments where motherhood is a social duty linked to status, when they can afford modern fertility treatment. Some women in low-income countries travel to Europe to receive treatment that is not available at home. I have encountered the case of a woman whose expensive trips unfortunately did not achieve the desired outcome, and her husband left her following their failed attempts. Whatever the social context and nature of pressure endured, the grief surrounding infertility is always difficult.

By redefining the boundaries of human reproduction, biomedicine wields not only a technical power, but also power over our value system and the limits of what is humanly acceptable. This is why we must question the relevance of medical intervention, justified in the name of "progress," along with their social impacts. As already mentioned, anthropologist David Le Breton reminds us that "the procedures made possible by biotechnologies require collective deliberation, a confrontation of viewpoints and values, political arbitration, and more."[7]

The medicalization process

A current in social sciences research has extensively documented the medicalization of natural processes, including childbirth, along with psychological and social phenomena. According to this current, some human experiences are treated as diseases, and problems that should be addressed and resolved socially are instead done so medically, for example through the use of pharmacology.[8]

Infertility problems are now quickly medicalized, using a host of increasingly invasive treatments. For instance, women are now advised to see a doctor after a year of unprotected sex if they are under 35, and after six months if they are over 35.[9] Many people are choosing to have children later in life, one factor that has contributed to the rise in infertility.[10] Today, nearly 16 percent of Canadian couples struggle with infertility, a rate that has doubled since the 1980s.[11] Without ignoring the significant increase of hypofertility and infertility, we are mainly concerned here with the impact of technical interventions used to combat these issues. These solutions offer good news, unless they occur within a social context that pressures the patients into hastily undergoing treatment, some of which are not without consequences, such as taking hormones. This is done quickly, when there is still doubt as to whether there is a real pathology, before the people concerned have enough time to reflect or receive adequate support to be able to express their wishes.

One woman I met while conducting research on childbirth recounted such an experience. She and her partner had been trying for a baby for ten years and had attempted various infertility treatments. Her partner wanted to continue treatments, but she found the process difficult. Then, just as she had begun to grieve her lost motherhood and decided to turn the page, she became pregnant naturally. She no longer wished to become a mother, and the ensuing events were not easy. Her partner left her after the birth, and the breakup was difficult. Her story is neither common nor representative. Yet it is informative. Social pressures can exacerbate the quest for fertility: though biomedicine offers treatment options, it also helps construct the quest. When pushed to the extreme, patients reach a point of no return and feel they no longer have the right to give up on fertility.

Surrogacy falls within the scope of this movement, as it is now an option for women who cannot carry a child (for example, if they have no uterus). The argument to legitimize the practice draws largely on cases where a woman provides the ovum, her partner provides the sperm, and the fertilized embryo is implanted into the uterus of a surrogate. This argument positions surrogacy as women helping women: one replacing the other only for pregnancy since the woman in demand can supply the genetic material.

These situations nonetheless instrumentalize the surrogate, since, as with other forms of the practice, she commits to carrying the child and then ceding it after birth. The fact that she transfers the child to its genetic mother does nothing to change the nature of the arrangement. The goal is still an exchange. Relinquishing the child makes the birth contractual by nature; the surrogate acts as a means to an end, a practice that is inconsistent with human dignity. Moreover, in the cases cited above, some surrogates come from low-income countries. Laura Harrison, associate professor at Minnesota State University, has conducted research on surrogate mothers in India. She documents how the "trope of women helping women" is used to naturalize and justify a practice that is fraught with inequality, despite affording surrogates a kind of "agency."[12]

It is therefore on the basis of "available means," that the desire for a child is maintained. A desire that can only be relinquished when it becomes impossible to satisfy. And, as we have seen, the limits of what is possible are constantly being redefined.

A few years ago, who would have thought that an ovum taken from a woman in Eastern Europe, fertilized in vitro by the sperm of a man living in North America, would create an embryo that, once frozen, would be shipped and implanted into the uterus of a woman (either in Africa or Asia) who, after giving birth to the child (often via C-section), would then give it to a company responsible for transferring it to the father?

All this, because someone wanted a child.

We need to question the social construction of this desire, managed by medicine. What role does medicine play in this context? Is it overstepping the limits of its own domain to invade the social sphere? By pushing back the right to mourn one's fertility to the extreme, and in participating in the use of women's bodies to solve a problem where no other solution exists, is medicine being ethical? The French research mission reports:

> By definition, surrogacy is not designed to have any of the commissioning parents carry the unborn child, which means that none of them is required to undergo the medical treatment necessary to allow pregnancy.[13]

This situation raises questions about the medical practice itself:

> When it comes to surrogacy, one of the "most striking ethical pitfalls" is that, in reality, it is the intended parents who engage the services of a care agency, which will then administer "care" to a third person—the surrogate.[14]

Is the desire for a child exacerbated by the offer of solutions to satisfy this desire, regardless of the means, ethical considerations, and social impacts? The psychoanalysts cited in the previous chapter also question the role of medicine when it comes to the wellbeing of the newborn, raising ethical concerns related to criteria of beneficence and non-maleficence:

> Prescribing IVF before surrogacy is equivalent to prescribing abandonment, and doctors are finding themselves in a paradoxical position in the face of this "abandonment prescription." They are aware of the deleterious effects early separation can have on mother and baby. They invented kangaroo care, skin-to-skin contact, and joint hospitalization to keep mothers and newborns together. They place the newborn on the mother's stomach at birth, or on her chest in cases of C-section, to help strengthen their bond. Are paediatricians and delivery doctors delirious to go to such lengths to preserve this bond of body and soul that we know today to be so important for a child's wellbeing? They have seen how these practices improve the odds of survival for premature babies, reduce the length of hospitalizations, the success of breastfeeding. How can they simultaneously prescribe abandonment? Whether he likes it or not, a genetic parent, at birth, is a stranger from the baby's point of view. Whether or not the parent has donated gametes, this is not the person the baby will recognize.[15]

Individualism: satisfying one's own desire

In terms of demand, the rise of individualism can make an unfulfilled desire for children impossible to live with, especially given that this desire can now be fulfilled by technology. But at what cost? French ethnologist Martine Segalen writes:

The longer the wait for a birth, the greater the desire for a child becomes, and technology seems to be in a position to satisfy this desire for those whom the California justice system has coined the name "intended parents." This wish is socially constructed, inscribed in the all-powerful contemporary individualism: the market organizes an offer of surrogacy with the click of a computer mouse that is dressed in emotive language.[16]

At the same time, we must ask ourselves: where is the support for women, men, or couples who feel distressed since fulfilling their dream seems impossible, unless they take the route that science has opened up? Such support could help them put the situation in perspective and explore healthier options.

Social infertility

Social infertility, or an inability to procreate due to social circumstances (i.e., being single or homosexual), is becoming a reproductive issue driven by advances in medicine. The search for solutions to the lack of the natural ability to give birth involves medicine. Wanting children thus motivates medical quest.

This is different from wanting to become a parent. In the above cases adoption is possible (not everywhere, of course, but it is an option in Canada), although the process is becoming more complicated and wait times are often very long. For some couples, however, adoption is ruled out anyway. What comes into play here, and is often the deciding factor, is what Françoise Héritier calls the "criterion of genetic truth in establishing filiation."[17] The wish is to "reproduce oneself," as Jacques Testart writes. And this requires the intervention of an expert. If the desire is for a child that embodies the genetic link, it may be necessary to find a woman to carry out the pregnancy.

Wanting children: a social construct

Pressure to have children persists. However, it does not necessarily target the same types of people or social groups. For example, gay couples are now a target market when it comes to reproductive services, as evidenced by the countless websites that offer suggestions on how to find a surrogate (in most cases for a fee).

Gay couples' reproductive status has been transformed in the wake of other social changes: homosexual relationships are now considered legitimate (in Canada, but not yet in many other countries) along with conjugal rights. This means their partnerships are subject to inheritance rights, among other things. It is a welcome shift, putting an end to discrimination that is unacceptable in any society that values equity.

Now that homosexuality has become normalized, to some extent, and our society recognizes gay marriage, the question is: can gay people become parents? In Canada, homosexual couples are allowed to adopt children based on the same criteria as heterosexual couples, and this is the case in other Western societies (although it is still the subject of some debate). But the lines are blurred once medical intervention, and the use of surrogacy, is sought for reproductive purposes.

This is what three French homosexuals wrote for the opening of the 2018 Estates General of Bioethics, a national bioethics debate:

> As homosexuals, we wish to take a stand against what we believe to be serious drifts, carried out in the name of extreme individualism, and against what is nothing more than an attempt to end the ban surrounding the reification of the human body [...] it is our duty as citizens and our moral responsibility to take a public stance in order to make an alternative and reasonable voice heard.

These men believe that access to medically assisted reproduction (for lesbian couples) and surrogacy (for gay male couples) is not a matter of equality, rights, or a fight against discrimination, since an inability to procreate is natural and proper to being a homosexual. For the authors, "fully assuming one's homosexuality also means accepting the associated limits." This argument is based on a notion of infertility as a natural condition, one that does not justify medical treatment since it is not a disease.

The three authors describe surrogacy as a reification of the woman's body and that of the child, which has become the object of a contractual transaction. They conclude that advances in technology do not necessarily represent moral progress, and they refuse to "serve as moral validation for an archaic and regressive vision of humanity, even in the name of freedom."[18]

And they are not alone. Julie Bindel and Gary Powell write:

> [...] our community is leading the way now in normalising, sanitising, and destigmatising this practice. Those who are proposing that surrogacy should be legalised, using the arguments of "gay rights" and equality, are subverting the core aims of the gay liberation movement, which is about dignity and respect for all, not abusing other people's rights.[19]

These testimonials touch on one of the central elements in the surrogacy debate: claiming the "right to a child," which is used to justify assisted reproductive technology. But there is no discrimination or injustice, only a difference in reproductive capacities. A man cannot conceive, carry, or birth a child, any more than a woman can supply the necessary sperm. The inability of gay couples to reproduce is not a disease. The proposed solutions involve using another human of a different sex. What, then, is the role of medicine if not to act as a go-between?

Questions also arise in cases of artificial insemination. We should wonder why so little importance is given to sperm donation, despite the fact that in surrogacy, it is considered essential enough to be prioritized over adoption. Why should this be? Because while adoption can make you a parent, it can't give you a genetic link to the child.

Right to a child

Recently, Quebec paediatrician Jean-François Chicoine acknowledged that "the desire for a child is legitimate, even inescapable, but it is all-consuming. In some cases, its tenacity is incompatible with human dignity." In an article published in *La Presse*, he noted:

> Since 2004, the decrease in the number of children newly adopted abroad was directly proportional to the increase in children conceived through surrogates abroad.[20] Like water, the desire for a child permeates. Morals, doctrines, and laws suit it, provided they do not hinder its evacuation and, beyond that, its relief, even its deviation: the right to a child.[21]

This notion is used to justify medical intervention and silence criticism of abuses associated with satisfying this desire. The role of medicine is thus transformed, making it responsible for righting wrongs, as Sylvie Epelboin points out:

> Advocating one's right to a child implies medicine has an egalitarian mission, no matter what is causing infertility: since there are solutions for women without ovaries (ovum donation), it would be unfair not to offer solutions for those without a uterus. The ovum retrieval process is onerous for the donor, but does not require the nine-month investment of pregnancy or the same health risks. Medicine cannot be held accountable for equal care in different pathologies, nor does it promise the same success for AHR in all types of infertility.[22]

Although the right to a child is often invoked, the report submitted to the HRC, cited in chapter 3, argues it does not exist and must be distinguished from the right to start a family and the right to have one's private and family life respected. In the conclusion of the collective work *Les incidences de la biomédecine sur la parenté (The Impacts of Biomedicine on Kinship)*, Françoise Dekeuwer-Défossez notes that it comes as no surprise that some invoke equal rights and discrimination (e.g., between homosexual and heterosexual couples) since the demand to use new medical techniques is based on individual rights. She stresses that "framing these egalitarian claims around the idea of discrimination does not help us find a fair solution. Instead, by refusing to acknowledge natural differences and by calling on society to fix them, we open the door to limitless human desires." She describes this situation as "the problem of setting legal limits to desires of all kinds..."[23]

What about the future?

The prospects of cloning and of creating an artificial uterus attest to just how far reproducing oneself could take us. Cloning reproduces an exact copy of oneself, and the artificial uterus allows to reproduce without the need for another human being. Is this what we want? Is this where a desire for children is leading, revised and corrected by a biomedicine that seeks to push the limits of technical achievements and whose "advancements" have no regard for the loss of humanity?

"In the biotechnological imagination," observes Sylviane Agasinski, "the child is nothing but a product made from crumbs: sperm, ova, uterus. What lies ahead if we disregard the dignity of both a person and their body?"[24]

A child of one's own? A child whose conception is only in one's own self-interest? Currently, children are seen less as a social contribution, less as a prolongation of the bloodline, and more as people in their own right. Yet we are now seeing a reactionary trend that places adults at the forefront of a quest for their own reproductive achievements.

Employing a technique that disregards the stages unique to human procreation represents a significant step backwards for otherness, since these stages hold the seeds of the parent-child bond. The human quality of the experience centred on otherness is then disavowed. Montreal journalist Agnès Gruda writes: "A Montreal-based hairstylist who had twins with help from a Bombay clinic uses striking language to sum up his experience: 'To me, a surrogate is like an oven.'"[25]

What are the medium- and long-term consequences of surrogacy if the practice is not collectively challenged? We must examine how the desire for a child is socially constructed. The sentiment is not pathological in itself, but it becomes so when the need to fulfil it comes at the price of human dignity.

Uncorrected Galleys

It is important to question the role of medicine, which should not be responsible for upholding the law or supporting the instrumentalization of women and the reification of children to satisfy a demand based on a desire. Among the ethical dilemmas surrogacy raises, let us recall both the principle of non-maleficence and respect for autonomy. As we know, depriving a child of its mother is likely to cause suffering. And, as previously noted in chapter 2, there are obvious issues with a surrogate's free and informed consent.

Researcher Françoise Dekeuwer-Défossez is unequivocal regarding the use of biomedicine and children's fate:

> Generally speaking, however, biomedicine makes it possible to meet the demands of adults without an ability or willingness to measure the implications on the lives of future children. Since the dawn of time, children have no doubt been at the mercy of their genitors. Abandonment and infanticide are as old as humanity, just as children's futures are closely related to the circumstances of their birth. The bastards of previous generations were deprived of filiation, like today's children born of surrogacy. We might have thought the voluntary and planned nature of biomedicine would have enabled us to consider the interests of unborn children in advance, thereby ensuring the best possible future for them. Yet even in the widespread and everyday use of common medical techniques, the child's best interests are scarcely considered.[26]

In short, surrogacy raises issues concerning gender relations, parent-child relations, and relations between social classes.

In the first case, the crucial role reproduction plays in gender relations has meant that as society has evolved, it has prompted an appeal to recognize shared contributions and responsibilities within the family. Reproduction that instrumentalizes the opposite sex leads to inequality and represents a marked step backwards. In the second, commissioning a child transforms the parental relationship into one that reifies the child. He or she becomes a being to be acquired and even purchased. This challenges parent-child relationships based on respect for the other; reproduction should, after all, be imprinted with human dignity. Finally, the inexorable commercialization of surrogacy, if not declared illicit, can only add to what has been previously observed and documented: it exploits disadvantaged women.

Relying on a surrogacy contract to satisfy a desire for a child does not signal the type of humane future that recent gains in human rights and freedoms seemed to promise.

Chapter 5

The Pieces of the Puzzle

Three dimensions of surrogacy must be examined more closely: the health of mother and child, the use of anthropological knowledge in the debate surrounding it, and the illusion that regulations can prevent women and children from being commodified.

The health of mother and child

Feminists have advocated humanization of birth care on the basis that pregnancy and childbirth are normal human events. They have also done so to minimize related risks thanks to preventive care, support during pregnancy, and medical interventions (when necessary and used wisely). Feminists have acted together with professionals including midwives, nurses, and doctors. Did their efforts bear fruit? Pregnancy has certainly become safer, but there is still much work to do to reduce the medicalization of the maternity experience.

When it comes to surrogacy, is there enough concern for the health of mothers and children, given the interventions necessitated by assisted reproductive methods? And are these methods in line with the orientations proposed by the women's health movement and those of the perinatal community?

The available information unfortunately indicates that priority is placed on efforts to produce a quality product for the commissioning parents. There is little concern for the health of the woman and her wellbeing vis-à-vis the "task" she is entrusted with. As for the child's health, it is desired, not to say required. If compromised, the child may be refused. Such cases have been documented.

Women who agree to act as surrogates commit to an experience that comes with associated risks. These are increased by the necessary technical interventions. Considering the circumstances of its birth, the child may also be exposed to more risk than would have occurred with a spontaneous pregnancy. The demand for a product here outweighs a concern for the health of mother and child. This holds true even in cases of surrogacy agreements between friends or family members, where pregnancies generally progress under better conditions than those in which surrogates wield little power and the buyers come from another continent.

Whatever the context, the situation is flawed from the start. Contracts create conditions that jeopardize the autonomy of the mother, who is the primary person affected by the pregnancy and childbirth experience, particularly with regard to the risks involved, insofar as these increased risks are not revealed.

Besides, what do we know of the risks? Information is lacking, since the contexts in which surrogates live while pregnant and later deliver their babies do not easily lend themselves to clinical or epidemiological research. To conduct these studies, the practice must be carried out legally and research methods must meet scientific criteria and secure financial and material support. These conditions are not often met.

The largest study to date of gestational surrogates and the only one to have evaluated antecedent spontaneous pregnancies achieved by the same women was recently conducted in the United States analyzing 124 women and 494 births. Of these, 352 were singleton live births, including 103 commissioned embryos and 249 spontaneously conceived embryos. The study confirms that commissioned births come with increased risk, and there was a significant difference in outcomes for surrogate and spontaneous pregnancies. Surrogate pregnancies more often resulted in twin pregnancies (33 percent versus 1 percent). Although rates of miscarriage and ectopic pregnancies were similar, adverse perinatal outcomes such as preterm birth, low birth weight, hypertension, maternal gestational diabetes, placenta previa, and the use of antibiotics during labour, along with rates of amniocentesis and C-section were higher in the case of commissioned births. The authors of the study conclude that assisted reproductive procedures may affect embryo quality and/or placentation.[1]

Another smaller study conducted in California in 2015 compared hospital costs incurred for surrogate births with those of naturally conceived births. Since hospital stays for surrogates are longer due to the higher incidence of C-sections, it follows that surrogate births are significantly more expensive (even discounting the cost of IVF procedures, artificial insemination, and embryo transfer). They are especially magnified in cases of triplets or multiple births, which are more common in surrogate births.[2] The results also confirm an increased risk associated with assisted reproductive techniques, which require a certain amount of manipulations.

So we know a little bit more. However, we will have to wait for further studies to complete the knowledge on the specific experience of surrogate mothers. The stakes are high, considering these pregnancies and deliveries are carefully planned. Is it acceptable to plan a pregnancy knowing it will involve more risks than a spontaneous one? How should medicine proceed in such circumstances?

One of the issues to consider is the more frequent use of C-sections in contract pregnancies. In fact, the surgery is often scheduled regardless of how healthy mother and child are at the time of delivery. It is even included in some surrogacy contracts for convenience purposes (i.e., to ensure the commissioning parents will be present or to avoid a long or complicated delivery).

Uncorrected Galleys

These abusive practices are indicative of how surrogacy fails to respect women's integrity. The high rates of C-sections in Quebec, the rest of Canada, and the United States undeniably contribute to trivializing the procedure and hinder a more judicious practice. It should be noted that this trivialization is not approved by those concerned with women's health, such as the World Health Organization or various medical associations. Here is what the Society of Obstetricians and Gynaecologists of Canada has to say:

> A C-section is a very common surgical procedure but still has associated risks. Babies born via C-section can have respiratory problems but these usually resolve quickly. The recovery time for the mother is longer and the risk of infection is greater compared to vaginal delivery. And, once there is a scar in your uterus, there are special considerations for your next labour. As with any surgery, there are complications that can arise. For example, the incision or the uterus can become infected, bleeding and blood clots are more likely, urinary tract infections can happen, and bowel function may be decreased.[3]

To sum up, C-sections should only be done when medically necessary. This curative intervention should be used electively only in cases where there are known risks involved (e.g., a risk of the uterus rupturing). Yet researcher Sheela Saravanan reports that in Indian clinics, before surrogacy for foreign commissioning parents was prohibited in 2016,[4] C-sections were systematic.

The website Surrogacy360.org warns of abusive C-sections. It urges future parents, who go through intermediaries to reach an agreement with a surrogate mother, to exercise caution in regard to three types of intervention: mandatory C-section, a procedure described as major abdominal surgery that slows and complicates recovery for surrogates, most of whom receive little or no care after delivery or at subsequent births; implanting multiple embryos into a single uterus to increase the chances of a healthy baby; and foetal reduction in cases of multifoetal pregnancies when the commissioning parents do not want more than one child.[5] These recommendations illustrate how the health of the surrogate mothers is of little concern when it comes to commercial practices.

Other risks threaten the health of surrogates, including side effects associated with certain hormone therapies that prepare their bodies for pregnancy.[6]

No pregnancy is risk-free, but other risks are added by the use of technical interventions involved in surrogacy. And the harmful conditions experienced by some surrogates present other risks, including a lack of postpartum care for mothers from underprivileged backgrounds who are left to fend for themselves once the baby has been given away.

Finally, surrogacy still involves a risk of maternal death. The October 2015 story of an American surrogate mother who died, along with the twins she was carrying, just days before a scheduled C-section was not widely reported. Journalists simply concluded that it would not have been the country's first maternal sur-

rogate death.[7] In January 2020, the death of a mother
of two, acting as a surrogate for the second time, was
also reported.[8]

The psychological risks associated with surrogacy are poorly documented. Sarah Jacob-Wagner, a
researcher for Quebec's Conseil du statut de la femme
(Council on the status of women), analyzed a number
of studies by grouping together the results according
to the various stages of childbirth: pregnancy, delivery,
postpartum.[9] These studies generally report positive
experiences, though they do mention some difficult
moments and sources of hesitation. The participants
do not report having any regrets. It is unclear, however,
as is the case with any study involving self-reporting,
whether women who experienced psychological difficulty simply chose not to disclose it.

Some studies have shown that in cases of surrogates
who come from underprivileged backgrounds, the
money earned makes up for any problems encountered.
As we have seen in chapter 2, some discourses sublimate
the act of giving away the child, no doubt making it
seem more acceptable. Some women, however, report
feeling humiliated by how the commissioning parents
treated them; others report feeling respected. A wide
range of experiences is possible, and information from
larger samples would help to better evaluate them. The
psychological experience of women throughout pregnancy, at the time of delivery, and after birth has always
been the poor relation of maternal health research. It

is not surprising that this is the case for contract pregnancies as well.

In short, the health of the mother and child is a critical issue when it comes to surrogacy. However, it is given little attention, revealing that the realization of a project takes precedence over the well-being of humans used to make it a reality.

Lessons from anthropology

By documenting a wide range of human and social experiences, the field of anthropology helps us better understand ourselves as humans and better grasp that diversity—including the various ways to frame human reproduction. Anthropology is particularly concerned with the rules of kinship and descent, which are at the heart of the organization of conjugality and families. This organization, rooted in dominant social relationships of class and gender, reflects the status of women and children. Knowledge collected across societies helps increase our understanding of current or past social practices.

Studies on our society provide keys to understanding the evolution of family and the changes observed in its organization. Anthropology can therefore help to grasp the meaning of social behaviours whether these are relationships between couples, between parents and children, or within extended families. For this reason, anthropology is particularly involved in the debates surrounding assisted reproduction.

But we should not absorb the knowledge we have acquired thus far without critical analysis. We now know about researcher bias and how researchers' own perspectives alter how they interpret what they observe—in their own society, but especially in others. This is why much of the research done by men examining the lived social realities of women across cultures has been called into question. These women may not even have been accessible to them due to tradition or belief systems. Before considering a foreign custom to be a model or a practice comparable to others, we must pay attention to how results have been interpreted.

Why should this concern us? Because the results of anthropological studies are often used out of context to justify or even promote certain social practices. It is less important in this case to revisit the research or its "objectivity" than it is to question how these studies are used.

Surrogacy advocates invoke the authority of anthropology to justify the instrumentalization of women, who are used to bear children without being considered their mothers, by citing similar practices observed elsewhere or previously. The information that some traditional practices may resemble surrogacy arrangements is problematic when used as an argument that this grants it some legitimacy. The adequacy between an alleged similarity and legitimacy is contestable.

Interpretations of this kind are particularly questionable when they involve descent. Illustrations are thus offered of societies where children are entrusted to someone other than their mother, taken in by a group of people, or considered to belong to a clan. It then seems to suggest, when it is not explicitly stated, that a surrogate "giving" a child to another couple falls within the scope of other known traditions. Yet these traditions cannot possibly be compared to todays', given the current context of technification of reproductive practices.

Not all anthropologists are united behind this type of comparative discourse. Maurice Godelier, an expert in the field of kinship, believes the changes prompted by assisted reproduction constitute a major shift:

> For the first time in human history, we need not two, but three bodies to make a child [...] This was unthinkable just a few decades ago: in the history of humanity, no myth, to my knowledge, has ever imagined such things![10]

The practice of surrogacy began towards the end of the 1970s. It cannot be compared to other methods, such as those observed by anthropologists in so-called traditional societies. The same goes for rules of descent: it is impossible to reproduce what happens in societies with a completely different economic and social organization, because to do so distorts the original context. We should instead examine Quebec's and Canada's own evolution, and that of similar societies, along with the processes we subscribe to as members of the international community. In this way we can study different methods of enriching our approach without losing the gains we have already made.

Uncorrected Galleys

The most ironic part of this line of reasoning (if it has been done before, we shouldn't be scared...) is that the most frequently cited examples throughout history are not drawn from anthropological research, but from the Bible! These are stories about the use of slaves or servants, such as Sarah, who gave her handmaid Hagar to Abraham so that she could bear him a son—a solution that requires neither anonymity nor technology.

Isn't there a more stimulating modern path than a return to the use of a servant or slave to have children? Surrogacy advocates don't seem to understand that by invoking these narratives, they demonstrate that these so-called similar practices do not respect basic human rights now recognized worldwide and sanctioned by many societies, including Western ones.

Another interpretation of anthropological observations sparks debate when it presents surrogacy as an innovative technique rich in opportunities that, to some extent, paves the way for the future. Martine Segalen notes:

> [...] research focuses on constructing new family ties between the parties involved, sometimes supporting the notion that this multi-parenting is part of the modernity of contemporary family life, and sometimes the notion that it is a question of radical innovations, or even an inevitable progress that will little by little establish itself in society.[11]

This view accuses opponents of surrogacy of being resistant to change and of rejecting "modernity" and (irreversible, some would argue) "progress." But before we deem these methods positive or lifesaving, we must ensure they do not represent setbacks on a human level nor on acquired rights.

The illusion of regulation

In recent years, a movement to promote surrogacy regulations, rather than banning the practice altogether in order to protect women and children, has gained much ground. In Quebec, the Family Law Advisory Committee chose this approach rather than maintaining the status quo, arguing "the practice has, does, and will continue to exist."[12] They argue it is the children who pay the price of surrogacy, and that it is necessary to break with past traditions of labelling them either *legitimate* or *illegitimate*. "There is no point denying the reality exists. Instead, we must recognize the practice and attempt to respond by enacting regulatory measures to protect all concerned parties."[13] The law often does legitimize situations once they have spread. But when this "reality" involves a lack of consensus, when it affects the status of women and children, and when it frames human reproduction in contractual terms, questions can be raised as to the appropriateness of such a course of action. Should we regulate in order to protect the concerned parties if this risks normalizing a practice that is wrong?

For legal experts, the current situation is far from ideal. Judges preside over cases where children will likely be penalized, by being considered illegitimate, because their so-called intended parents commissioned women from low-income countries and now want these children to be recognized as their own. Judges must act in the best interests of the child. We have seen that their interpretation can lead judges to decide that the "intended" parents are best placed to act as family to the child since they have commissioned the birth, have a genetic link (the father), and that the child does not have a mother anyway. This is how commissioning parents succeed!

The Family Law Advisory Committee outlines the following principles:

> 1) Regardless of the mixed feelings that the parental project involving the use of a surrogate mother may arouse in us, the resulting child must not be penalized in any manner from the actions committed by the parties involved; it is about its interest and respecting its rights; 2) Regardless of their motivations, women who agree to act as surrogate mothers cannot be abandoned to their fate; their protection and respect for their dignity are at stake.[14]

Although the Committee acknowledges it is uncomfortable with the practice of surrogacy, it proposes guidelines and a legal framework addressing, among others, the consent of the surrogate mother, a particularly contentious issue. It recognizes the surrogate's right to decide to keep the child after giving birth, thus hoping to avoid regulating the instrumentalization of a human being. As for the rest, the principles invoke the shared values concerned with the child's best interests and respect for the mother's dignity.

Three arguments can be used to oppose the adoption of a legal framework and maintain the Civil Code's current status that does not recognize surrogacy contracts: 1) a socially illegitimate process should never be legalized, and regulation does not make it legitimate; 2) acting in the child's best interests can be interpreted differently from the way the Committee report defines it; and 3) in an economy such as ours, it is unrealistic to ignore the fact that granting a legitimate status to surrogacy will inevitably lead to its commercialization in the short or medium term.

Surrogacy's social illegitimacy

Surrogacy challenges women's rights, specifically their dignity as humans; a human can never be a means to an end. Surrogacy is not socially legitimate, especially considering how much women have fought for centuries—particularly since the 19th century—to be recognized as persons in their own right, capable of performing the same functions as a man and no more confined to reproductive roles (childbirth, caregiving, domestic work). And the gains are evident. Women have entered the public domain and hold positions of authority at societal levels. Legalizing a practice that subjects some of them to fulfilling a reproductive role for the sole purpose of satisfying sponsors is unacceptable in this context; suggesting that regulation would better protect these women changes nothing in this respect.

People who believe that regulation will better protect surrogates should not let their good intentions overshadow the fact that these women often come from underprivileged backgrounds and low-income countries. This reality challenges us far beyond possible arrangements and reveals what is at the heart of the process: exploiting other human beings to achieve a personal goal. Inequality is written into the nature of surrogacy, and legally regulating a practice that is based on an unequal power dynamic cannot validate it.

Are there commissioning parents in demand for surrogates (we're not talking about intermediaries and facilitators here)? It doesn't matter. They are not dependent upon supply. They can always seek a woman elsewhere. Once the contract has been signed, the woman is clearly subordinate: she has committed to an experience that will require both mind and body, and she is doing it not for herself, but for others. She should be protected, but from what? Abuse? We must rather condemn a practice that is wrapped in an illusory, manipulative, and in some cases fraudulent discourse that manages to convince the woman to act as a tool to serve others. How can we spare her this status inherent to the contract, if not by declaring it null and void?

The danger here is not the lack of regulation around an unacceptable practice; instead, the real danger is that by regulating the practice, we deem it acceptable.

Uncorrected Galleys

The legal provision affirming surrogacy contracts
to be null (article 541 of the Civil Code) could still be
effective. Some would claim that lax regulatory policies
make it easy to bend the law, as sometimes happens.
But for the law to do its job, it must be applied with
zero tolerance. This means that commissioning parents
should not be able to rely on a *fait accompli*, as they now
do, returning from elsewhere with a child a judge feels
obligated to acknowledge as legally their own. Judges
could decide otherwise and entrust the child to parents
who respect and uphold the law. This may seem like a
drastic solution, but if the Civil Code deems surrogacy
contracts null, it can only be because society does not
consider the practice to be acceptable.

Nevertheless, we must not delude ourselves; the
situation in Quebec is complex because its position on
surrogacy differs from the 2004 decision adopted by
Canada to recognize the practice—which is confus-
ing, to say the least, when we observe the reality. Yet
giving in and conforming to the Canadian position
will not help the situation. It will make it extremely
difficult to limit the development of commercial practices that already exist in Canada, that is reproductive
tourism to other countries and that of foreign couples
to Quebec. Why? Because social discord surrounding surrogacy means critics want it strictly regulated.
This is what is happening with Family Law Advisory
Committee proposals. Reassured that surrogacy practices are now allowed at home, many commissioning

Uncorrected Galleys

parents will go elsewhere, still preferring more flexible rules.

The child's best interests

Could a surrogacy practice be specifically designed to protect women and children? Even in this case, respecting the child's human dignity remains an issue. We cannot stress enough that children are not commodities and have rights: to know where they come from and live with the people who gave them life, whenever possible. Depriving a child of this opportunity should not be arranged through a contract.

Those who, in a manner of speaking, take the child hostage (after it has been abandoned by its mother) are named in the contract as the child's only guardians. Yet they should not be in the right. Couples that travel to countries with more permissive laws should be neither gratified nor absolved of their actions.

Quebec should not model itself on any of the countries that allow surrogacy arrangements. One of the worst examples comes from the United States; other cases often involve countries where respect for human rights is a pipe dream. We must look elsewhere for inspiration.

No matter what the terms of a surrogacy contract are, children still lose out on a primary relationship and a part of their origin story. The fact that children and their futures are so often overlooked in the debate should raise the alarm. They become an object of desire

Uncorrected Galleys

with no voice, their fate sealed in a contract that is legal (acknowledging a separation from the mother) or illegal. And as we now know, commissioning parents can always force the hand of the law if necessary—supposedly in the name of the child's best interests.

Since the United Nations was founded, efforts have been made to ensure children are not psychologically, physically, or socially abused or exploited. Given how surrogacy stirs up debate around the child's wellbeing, these remain fundamental principles. The report submitted to the HRC considered the use of surrogacy could be likened to the sale of a child. This is what we know of the existing "reality." Must we legitimize the situation in order to regulate it, which essentially means justifying surrogacy under certain conditions? Absolutely not. The risks to children are far too great.

Inevitable fallouts

Arguments that support an "altruistic" model to counter rights abuses merely confuse the issue. In Quebec, there has been a movement to recognize and regulate only this type of surrogacy, implying that in this form, surrogacy is acceptable. But we must not forget that this "friendlier" model does not guarantee the child will know its mother.

What does "altruistic" actually mean in these circumstances? Essentially, that it is free! The rest is anecdotal. In other words, opening the door to "altruistic" surrogacy (as Canada has done) only means the arrangement is legal provided the surrogate is not paid. To believe this process will remain an act of pure generosity, once legalized and undertaken within a framework of capitalism, is to greatly underestimate the human imagination.

It is unrealistic to think that the theoretical model of "altruistic" pregnancy will translate as such in practice, once the validity of the contracts is recognized. This model, exercised within families or between close relations, cannot be projected to a larger scale without being redefined according to society's prevailing norms. This becomes evident as Canada's reproductive industry grows and intermediaries are recognizing surrogacy as a gold mine. Companies such as Canadian Fertility Consulting, discussed in chapter 1, who claim to operate as "altruistic" providers do not hide the fact that they are ready for commercialization. Credulity in the face of such knowledge has no place. Human reproduction has been taken hostage by merchants hiding behind a discourse of love and giving. If businesses did not find profit in this, why would they exist?

The Health Canada consultation conducted in the summer of 2017 provides a good example of the ambiguity that surrounds free surrogacy services. The consultation focused on defining policy and regulations and was aimed specifically at the reimbursement of expenses incurred (both donors and surrogates). One proposal was prepared by the CSA Group (Canadian Standards Association) and circulated by Health Canada, as an example. The items eligible for reimbursement covered almost everything, with some items that could be considered as a form of remuneration. Health Canada then consulted stakeholders in the assisted reproduction industry—with specific references to surrogate mothers—and returned with a draft proposal in October 2018.

This step consolidates the status of surrogacy in order to make it perfectly legitimate across Canada, with practical information on how to compensate legally a surrogate mother. So far, Health Canada had refrained from estimating the costs associated with pregnancy. By calculating related costs, pregnancy can be assessed in financial terms. We already know that pregnancy generates expenses (e.g., maternity clothes), but this is different from establishing quantifiable methods for reimbursing pregnancy-related expenses that are the responsibility of commissioning parents. Though the value of the calculation changes according to the contract terms, it lays the foundation for commodification. Health Canada's October 2018 project was born from an entrepreneurial vision and clearly addresses reproductive intermediaries and agencies. The obvious objective is to enable them to operate legally. Hard to beat as a measure to support the industry's development.[15]

Such realities force us to think. We must reimagine a way to end surrogacy by developing alternative paths for those who wish to become parents.

Conclusion

We still have much to study when it comes to the complex experience of motherhood. What we know so far also urges us to take much bolder action to protect children, who don't have any say on an existence arising from a contract. In the name of human values, these children must be welcomed in the best possible conditions in which to grow and thrive. What's more, we need to re-examine current approaches and explore other ways to take care of children by knowing how to meet their needs, while acknowledging the wishes of adults who want to become parents but are unable to procreate. In addition to these collective efforts, we must find a way to end the practice of surrogacy, as evidenced by the arguments laid out in the preceding chapters.

The nature of the demand

The paragraph below is taken from Quebec's Family Law Advisory Committee report concerning people struggling to become parents:

Committee members have observed an inexorable reality. Like it or not, the desire for a child is so powerful that it will justify, in the minds of those who feel it, the use of all forms of assisted procreation, even gestation (surrogate mother), regardless of the legality of the arrangements or the content of the penalties that will be attached to them.[1]

These words sound like an admission of powerlessness. When desire becomes an obsession, it causes suffering. Yet efforts to relieve this suffering should not legitimate a practice that forces us to reject our collective values. Instead, we must do everything in our power to avoid the construction of an unacceptable model of reproduction which some will unduly take advantage of. We must prevent trapping people who are suffering in a quest that many seek to exploit.

Many adults hoping to start a family are unable to have children naturally, but their demand should not be invariably answered by a medical intervention. Instead, it should be addressed in a different manner. We should analyze existing options and channels that facilitate parenthood, and at the same time make sincere efforts to support innovation. This requires political will, including a readiness to attack the cultural and social representations that feed the construction of the desire to have a child.

We have discussed the cultural evolution that has led to what is now called "the desire for a child," as well as how infertility has transitioned from a medical diagnosis to one that can be primarily social in nature. The number of situations in which we see people, with this desire, claiming it justifies surrogacy, thus exceeds the number of situations of infertility previously recorded.

Above all, we must not judge from the outset these people who, for the most part, have been led to consider that they can have a child because medicine makes it possible today. Contrary to the ideas peddled by the increasing number of surrogacy advocates and life merchants, however, the fundamentally human dimension of surrogacy sets it apart from any other technique. We must explore other options. If we rule out the surrogacy "solution," which is harmful, what alternatives can be considered?

We have much to learn and retain from what researchers can tell us about what was happening in the past and what is happening elsewhere. All of this knowledge, however, needs to be considered in today's context. In the aftermath of World War II, international organizations were founded to examine our human and social relationships. Central to these debates is the issue of rights and freedoms. Huge gains have been made, although they are not enough. We need to explore more "modern" forms of parenthood based on these achievements.

Why don't we side with children? What if the guiding principle of our reflections was to meet the needs of those already born?

Adoption exists, of course, but it has become more difficult in recent years because fewer children are now orphaned in Western countries, which, by the way, we should be happy about. International adoption has also become more complicated with longer wait times, requirements that conflict with our way of life. Yet there are many children who are still in need of parents. Let's not forget that adoption is not about fulfilling the needs of an adult, but about finding a family for a child in need. More energy should be put into supporting potential parents and connecting them with children. We should devote as much energy to these initiatives as we do to assisting and supporting natural parents, especially considering how difficult adoption can be.

Using a surrogate from an underprivileged country is not consistent with the Canadian and Quebec values of human dignity and gender equality. These values are, however, consistent with welcoming children from such a country where conditions make it impossible for them to receive an education, or children born into conflict zones who may be terrorized, hurt, or even killed. Not enough efforts are made in this regard, and adults able to take in these children do not find adequate support. This must change. The work accomplished at the international level should serve as a starting point to go further in respecting children's rights by enabling them to find a family, while distancing from the sale of children—a risk inherent to surrogacy.

We can also do a better job of looking after children born in Canada who have developmental, behavioural, or other issues. It is no secret that caring for these children presents specific challenges, and that taking them in is not the same as welcoming a newborn. Yet it can be a social contribution that is highly rewarding for the adults who commit themselves to it, and it provides children with a home enabling them to grow up in an environment offering a better chance of success. Again, it takes true political will to ensure that our most vulnerable children—those who lack parental guidance—can grow up in a family that will provide them with stability.

And we can undoubtedly develop other approaches. A couple (two women) I knew wanted to experience motherhood without turning to assisted reproductive technology, so they decided to become "extra" parents for children who needed support. They found their role as educators to be very rewarding, and they developed a bond with the children. I knew another couple that opened their home to two teenagers who allowed themselves to be parented by other adults, while still in contact with their mother who was unable to raise them. The couple had to dramatically alter their lifestyle to provide the children with constant support. Although they were older, they still needed the security of loving adults who believed in their potential.

These are both anecdotes, but they illustrate how the role of a parent can take many forms. Prioritizing the needs of a child over the needs of an adult opens vast possibilities for getting involved in their care and education.

Such choices, however, require abandoning the idea of making a baby; they appeal to different values than the quest to reproduce at any cost.

Why not draw inspiration from the results of studies that allow us to appreciate human diversity in order to support "modern" efforts to care for our children from a perspective of human dignity? How can the world view that has driven the societies that preceded us or that exist elsewhere inspire us? Why not learn from traditional practices of child circulation and draw on a model of collective responsibility for the development of children, instead of taking the practice out of context to justify making motherless children?

From the family law perspective, we could focus on ways to develop different parenting arrangements that respect everyone's rights, instead of regulating what undeniably entails a human cost. By analyzing children's diverse circumstances and needs, we can identify new models of "child circulation" for those lacking parental support. To do so, we must examine how best to support children and future parents, and we must encourage socially acceptable forms of regulation. It is a vast terrain, but it is better to build from the ground up than to try to fix the broken pieces since some are beyond repair.

Abolishing surrogacy internationally

I am not alone in rejecting the argument that if surrogacy exists, it must be regulated to protect women, children, and potential parents. Other countries that have relied on this logic have witnessed an increase in the national demand for surrogacy. With supply proving insufficient to meet it, adults are going across borders where they are, most often, supported by shrewd for-profit agencies that are both eager to boost revenue and able to circumvent many laws.

This must be resisted.[2] The best way forward is an international ban on surrogacy and it is possible. Moreover, this solution cannot be rejected on the grounds that it opposes advances in science, one argument used to criticize those who oppose genetics research. The issues should not be conflated; this is about prohibiting a practice that violates human rights.

Countries that consider surrogacy to be an attack on human dignity must unite behind a movement to gradually put an end to women's exploitation and the baby-on-demand phenomenon worldwide. Shouldn't *jus cogens*, the fundamental human rights of children, be invoked at the level of international law, since through surrogacy they become "products of exchange," whereas they should never be the subject of trade, sale, or exchange? Other international mechanisms, including conventions that were specifically established to protect children, can be brought to bear. Many countries, dictatorships aside, currently prohibit surrogacy and many disadvantaged nations like India, after having been lax, have become more severe or outright closed down.

Light must be shed on existing practices and the ways in which traders in human reproduction benefit. Their strategies, which play to women's emotions and the pseudo-advantages of "renting out" their wombs, have to be exposed. The entire industry is feeding an unbridled desire to have children at all costs and is developing with no concern for the child's wellbeing.

International alliances led by feminists, which have been joined by various groups, already exist. Stop Surrogacy Now represents organizations and individuals from eighteen countries. The recently created International Coalition for the Abolition of Surrogate Motherhood (ICASM) brings together associations from eight countries. These organizations, among other activities, share information about surrogacy in different forums. Other actors in the fields of ethics, legal sciences, health sciences, social sciences, philosophy, children's rights and more, are working hard to make known the meaning of surrogacy and its consequences.

Canada and Quebec must decide which models used elsewhere best suit their own contexts. Currently, we have closer political and social ties to countries that prohibit surrogacy. In the United States, for example, several states still uphold the death penalty, the right to bear arms takes precedence over the protection of life, and paid maternity leave does not exist. When it comes to reproductive practices, is this the example we want to follow? Don't our values fall more in line with European countries, the majority of which have outlawed surrogacy?

Quebec is a territory within Canada and does not recognize surrogacy. Nothing prevents it from maintaining this position. Many of its current social policies already set it apart from the rest of the country. Take, for example, programs in early childhood, preventive leave for women who are pregnant or breastfeeding, and parental leave policies. The rest of Canada should rethink its position. Current trends point to an insidious acceptance of surrogacy's commercialization, though on a political level, Canada continues to claim itself a champion of human rights.

What now?

Proposals made by Quebec's Family Law Advisory Committee cite concern for the child as the reason they support regulation over maintaining the current nullity of contracts.

And yet, it would be possible for the courts to protect children brought to Canada whose parents have defied the spirit of Quebec's Civil Code by using a foreign surrogate. French legal experts have proposed ways to protect these children without sanctioning the practice or allowing the parents, not being penalized, to be encouraged to search for options abroad. Why not do the same in Quebec?

Quebec's values are in line with the refusal to recognise the validity of a contract giving access to a child even before conception. Will some people attempt to circumvent the legislation? Without a doubt! But in these cases, we can consider their status as parents to be socially illegitimate. Legal instruments need to be devised so that the children of offending parents are not the ones labelled illegitimate. They didn't ask to be born, and we must protect them. Illegitimate parents should be treated as such, and future policies must ensure more children are not placed in the same situation.

Final thoughts

I tend to compare surrogacy to environmental issues.

There are similarities on several levels. First, both situations are evolving rapidly. Environmental problems attributed to human action are relatively recent and stem from activities considered evidence of "progress" and economic growth. Surrogacy is an even more recent development whose origins lie in the representation of the human body as a machine that has driven medical research and innovation. Within this narrative, the body is fragmented and dissociated from psychological and social experiences. In the case of contract maternity, an attempt is made to give precedence to such a conception.

The thread of "progress" is central to both issues, which can be problematic: anything can be justified in the name of the "advancement" of mankind. In both cases, we rely on our ability to adapt and adjust in order to minimize the consequences of "harmful side effects." This makes it possible to avoid curbing behaviour that is injurious to the planet or to endorse an equally injurious reproductive practice. We try to convince ourselves that humans will learn to adapt to a ravaged planet, just as children will learn to adapt to new forms of parenthood (that may benefit certain adults, not them).

Both issues are responsible for blatant injustices. Economic development has evolved against a backdrop of growing inequality; rich countries are profiting from the poorest countries and from the most impoverished populations. Those left out of this development are to be found in the poorest countries. As for medically assisted reproduction and more specifically surrogacy, it is expanding, thanks to poorer women who are less fortunate than those men and women who take control of their reproductive potential—and their lives—for nine months.

Then there is an attitude of resignation in the face of the facts. Environmental concerns seem to prompt little engagement, even though many people, and specifically the younger generations, devote much energy to the cause. Worries over the future of our planet elicit few behavioural changes, as if the fight were futile. Similarly, the rapid increase in surrogacy has prompted many to give up. Though legal experts may disapprove, they feel powerless and instead opt for a harm reduction approach—an option that is perfectly valid in some spheres, but which takes on a whole new meaning in matters of human dignity.

A comparison of these two evolutions, both leading to an impasse, underlies my reflection on the rhetoric aimed at rallying support for the use of surrogacy. Developed very rapidly, it is seen as progress, yet the practice takes us back to an era where women and children were bereft of human rights.

Believing regulation will stamp out surrogacy's detrimental effects is no better than believing the planet will survive even if we do nothing concrete to protect the environment. In both cases, certain practices that are based on individualistic values and that prioritize individual freedoms must be ended.

True freedom is human freedom. It is exercised with an awareness of others and of the importance of preserving social ties and solidarity. Exercising human freedom is based on respect for all women, all men, and all children.

Notes

Foreword.

1. Some might claim that this debate occurred in Canada during the Royal Commission on New Reproductive Technologies, established in 1989, whose 1993 report led to a 2004 law. The context at that time was very different from that of today, and numerous resignations revealed that the Commission's debates were confrontational in nature.

2. SQ 2017, c 12.

Introduction

1. Incest taboo: "The prohibition of incest relates to the social rule that forbids sexual (rather than matrimonial) relations between individuals because of existing family ties (by blood or alliance)." Encyclopédie universalis, https://www.universalis.fr/encyclopedie/prohibition-de-l-inceste/ [trans.]; The term "type two incest" was coined by anthropologist Françoise Héritier and refers to sharing a sexual partner by blood relations of the same sex. She developed this concept in *Les deux sœurs et leur mère. Anthropologie de l'inceste* (Paris: Odile Jacob, 1994).

2. Enric Porqueres i Gené, "Corps relationnel, inceste et parenté aux temps de la génétique globalisée," *Ethnologie française* 167, 2017, p. 520 [trans.].

3. In 2013, Sheela Saravanan noted that in the United States, the surrogate mothers received about 35 percent of the amount paid, while in India this number was 10–15 percent. Sheela Saravanan,

"An ethnomethodological approach to examine exploitation in the context of capacity, trust and experience of commercial surrogacy in India," *Philosophy, Ethics and Humanities in Medicine*, 2013, 8:10.

4. Civil Code of Quebec, CQLR c CCQ-1991, c. 64, art 541, as amended by SQ 2002, c. 6, s 30.

5. The English version of the act uses the term "pay consideration" which refers to remuneration as well as to other forms of compensation.

6. Assisted Human Reproduction Act, S.C. 2004, c. 2, art 3.

7. Ibid, art 6 (4).

8. Ibid, art 6 (1).

9. Ibid, art 6 (2).

10. Ibid, art 6 (3).

11. Toward a strengthened *Assisted Human Reproduction Act*: A Consultation with Canadians on Key Policy Proposals, July 2017; For stakeholders of the Assisted Human Reproduction industry: Survey of Assisted Human Reproduction sector stakeholders affected by Health Canada's proposal to develop regulations under the *Assisted Human Reproduction Act*, November 2017.

12. Dib, Lina, "Un député veut décriminaliser les grossesses payées," *Le Nouvelliste*, 27 mars 2018, https://lenouvelliste.ca/actualites/le-fil-groupe-capitales-medias/un-depute-veut-decriminaliser-les-grossesses-payees-0fc3785bbdf-0f586b6e4d71d46517e39.

13. https://www.canadainternational.gc.ca/thailand-thailande/consular_services_consulaires/Surrogacy_Substitution.aspx-?lang=eng, accessed February 2020.

14. Vanessa Gruben, Alana Cattapan and Angela Cameron (eds), *Surrogacy in Canada, Critical Perspectives in Law and Policy*, Toronto, Irwin Law, 2018. This collective work released in late 2018 addresses various issues within the Canadian context. I authored the Afterword entitled *Legitimizing Surrogacy —_A Social Setback*.

15. https://www.canamcryo.com/en/eggs-donor-catalogue. It is possible to choose the characteristics of the donor (ethnicity, eye and hair color, height, etc.). Once a woman is chosen, she is added to the "cart," accessed February 2020.

16. My emphasis.

17. Sent by email on June 11, 2018, and signed by the Health Products Compliance Program, Regulatory Operations and Regions Branch, Health Canada.

18. Alison Motluk, "After pleading guilty for paying surrogates, business is booming for this fertility matchmaker," *The Globe and Mail*, February 28, 2016, updated May 16, 2018, https://www.theglobeandmail.com/life/health-and-fitness/health/business-is-booming-for-fertility-matchmaker-leia-swanberg/article28930242/.

19. On this issue: Diane Beeson, Marcy Darnovsky and Abby Lippman, "What's in a name? Variations in terminology of third-party reproduction, *Reproductive BioMedicine Online*, 2015, p. 805-814

20. Human Rights Council (HRC), *Report of the Special Rapporteur on the sale and sexual exploitation of children, including child prostitution, child pornography and other child sexual abuse material*, 37th session, February 26 – March 23, article 57, p. 14: (A/HRC/37/60) https://ap.ohchr.org/documents/dpage_e.aspx?m=102 accessed February 2020.

21. "What happens in the rhetoric of altruistic surrogacy is that it subversively accustoms people to seeing pregnancy as something a woman can lend to others—if she is not selling it," Kajsa Ekis Ekman in *Being and Being Bought: Prostitution, Surrogacy and the Split Self*, cited in Catherine Lynch, "Ethical Case for Abolishing all Forms of Surrogacy," *SundayGuardian Live*, October 28, 2017, https://www.sundayguardianlive.com/lifestyle/11380-ethical-case-abolishing-all-forms-surrogacy.

22. "Surrogacy" is the most common term used in English. For this reason, we use it in this essay, as we use "surrogate." Sometimes we write "surrogate mothers," as a reminder they are mothers. In French, we always prefer "the use of mothers *carrying*," which does not have a satisfying equivalent in English.

23. Jérôme Courduriès, "Ce que fabrique la gestation pour autrui." *Journal des anthropologues*, 2016, p. 54 [trans.].

Uncorrected Galleys

24. Laurent S. Barry et al., Glossaire de la parenté, *L'HOMME*, 154-155, 2000, p. 729. Accessible at https://journals.openedition.org/lhomme/58 [trans.].

25. Ibid, p. 724.

26. Renée Joyal, "Parenté, parentalité et filiation. Des questions cruciales pour l'avenir de nos enfants et de nos sociétés," *Enfances, familles, générations. Évolution des normes juridiques et nouvelles formes de régulation de la famille: regards croisés sur le couple et l'enfant*, Renée Joyal and Alain Roy (dir.), no. 5, 2006, p. 7 [trans.].

27. CCQ-1991, c. 64, art 655.

28. This system refers to "forms of belonging of the child to adults who are defined as his parents according to the kinship system," Maurice Godelier, "Systèmes de parenté et formes de famille," *Recherches de Science Religieuse* Vol. 102, no. 3, 2014, p. 357-372, p. 360 [trans.].

29. Laurent S. Barry, et al., op. cit., p. 725.

30. Ibid, p. 726.

31. Justice Québec: https://www.justice.gouv.qc.ca/en/couples-and-families/parenthood/filiation/, accessed October 2018.

32. Renée Joyal, op. cit., p. 5.

Chapter 1. Surrogacy's Emergence, Development, and International Expansion

1. The first in vitro baby, Louise Brown, was born in England. It doubtless would have happened on American soil if it hadn't been for the moratorium on research on in vitro fertilization imposed by the U.S. government.

2. The "right to child" claim will be addressed in Chapter 4.

3. Encyclopedia Universalis, https://universalis.fr/encyclopedie/individualisme/, accessed June 2018 [trans.].

4. First child, 29, second 31.2 and third, 32.6. Institut de la statistique du Québec, http://www.stat.gouv.qc.ca/statistiques/population-demographie/naissance-fecondite/403.htm, accessed June 2018.

5. Gilles Houle and Roch Hurtubise, "Parler de faire des enfants, une question vitale." *Recherches sociographiques,* 32(3), 1991, p. 412 [trans.].

6. Jacques Testart, *Faire des enfants demain,* Paris, Seuil, 2014.

7. Hospital insurance was adopted in Quebec in 1960, accelerating the shift from the home birth to the hospital birth. This led to developments in obstetrical interventions which subsequently multiplied, especially once health insurance was introduced in 1970.

8. Canadian Institute for Health Information (CIHI), Health Indicators Interactive Tools, https://yourhealthsystem.cihi.ca/epub/search.jspa?href=https%3A//yourhealthsystem.cihi.ca/epub/SearchServlet, accessed February 2020.

9. Françoise Héritier, *Masculin/Féminin,* tome I, *La pensée de la différence,* Paris, Éditions Odile Jacob, 1996, p. 284. [trans.].

10. Françoise Héritier, "La filiation, état social," *La revue lacanienne,* vol. 3 n° 8, 2010, p. 35. [trans.].

11. Sylvie Martin, *Le désenfantement du monde,* Montréal, Liber, 2011, p. 206 [trans.].

12. Simone de Beauvoir, *Le deuxième sexe,* Paris, Gallimard, 1970.

13. Despite recent improvements, many careers still require such choices. This reality can account for the delay in motherhood and may explain certain suggestions aimed at women (freezing their ova if they wish to put off motherhood while advancing their career): Marcia C. Inhorn, "Women, Consider Freezing your Eggs," *CNN.com,* 2013, https://www.cnn.com/2013/04/09/opinion/inhorn-egg-freezing/index.html, accessed November 2018; see also Procrea clinic advertisements (Ontario, Montreal, Quebec City), https://procrea.ca/fertility-treatment-options/egg-freezing/, accessed November 2018.

14. Maria De Koninck, "Dévalorisation et déqualification du rôle maternel: est-ce la faute des féministes?" Speech delivered at the symposium *Marcher sur des oeufs – Certains enjeux du féminisme aujourd'hui,* organized by the Conseil du statut de la femme, 1998 [trans.]. Also on the theme: Myriam Coulombe-Pontbriand,

"Maternité et liberté. Malaise du féminisme moderne, *Argument*, vol. 2, n° 10, 2008, http://www.revueargument.ca/.

15. Paris, Fayard, 2004.

16. Jean-Hugues Déchaux, "Les défis des nouvelles techniques de reproduction: comment la parenté entre en politique," in Brigitte Feuillet-Liger and Maria-Claudia Crespo-Brauner (dir.), *Les incidences de la biomédicine sur la parenté*, Brussels, Bruylant, 2014, p. 324 [trans.].

17. Reading her work invalidates how some would make use of it by interpreting the famous "one is not born, but rather becomes, a woman" as a denial of biological sex in order to replace it with the social construct of gender.

18. Definition according to Statistics Canada, http://www23.statcan.gc.ca/imdb/p3Var.pl?Function=DEC&Id=410445 accessed October 2018.

19. Joan W. Scott, "Gender: A Useful Category of Historical Analysis," *The American Historical Review*, vol. 91 no. 5, 1988, p. 1053-1075.

20. Jérôme Courduriès, "La gestation pour autrui, faire naître des pères et des mères," in Isabelle Côté, Kevin Lavoie, Kevin and Jérôme Courduriès (dir.), *Perspectives internationales sur la gestation pour autrui, Expériences des personnes concernées et contextes d'action*, Québec, Presses de l'Université du Québec, 2018, p. 138 [trans.].

21. And many other dimensions of modern life. Céline Lafontaine's book, *Le corps marché, La marchandisation de la vie humaine à l'ère de la bioéconomie* (The Body Market: The commodification of human life in the era of the bioeconomy), Paris, Seuil, 2014 is an excellent source of information to understand the development of the "economy of the living", along with its consequences on humans.

22. Françoise Dekeuwer-Défossez, "Réflexions conclusives," in Brigitte Feuillet-Liger and Maria-Claudia Crespo-Brauner, op. cit., p. 360 [trans.].

23. https://www.ohchr.org/EN/ProfessionalInterest/Pages/Slavery Convention.aspx.

24. Marie-Anne Frison-Roche, "Prohibition de la GPA convergence absolue entre droits des femmes et droits des enfants," May 2, 2016, http://mafr.fr/fr/article/denoncer-la-strategie-des-industriels-de-lhumain-c/, accessed October 2018. [trans.].

25. See note 14.

26. HRC, op. cit., article 15, p. 5.

27. Ibid, article 14, p. 4-5.

28. Cambodia police raid child surrogacy ring involving 33 surrogate mothers, July 23, 2018, Génèthique, http://www.genethique.org/en/cambodia-police-raid-child-surrogacy-ring-involving-33-surrogate-mothers-70121.html#.Xl7kCErCo2w.

29. South-East Asia, a real reproduction supply chain for Chinese couples, July 12, 2018, Généthique, http://www.genethique.org/en/south-east-asia-real-reproduction-supply-chain-chinese-couples-70069.html#.Xl7GnErCo2w

30. https://surrogacy360.org/considering-surrogacy/current-law/, accessed September 2018.

31. Françoise Dekeuwer-Défossez, op. cit., p. 361 [trans.].

32. https://www.creativefamilyconnections.com/us-surrogacy-law-map, accessed February 2020.

33. Robert Cribb and Emma Jarratt, "How Canada is becoming a key player in global surrogacy," *The Star,* June 25, 2016, https://www.thestar.com/news/world/2016/06/25/how-canada-is-becoming-a-key-player-in-global-surrogacy.html, accessed September 2018.

34. HRC, op. cit., article 29, p. 9.

35. "Lok Sabha passes Surrogacy (Regulation) Bill 2016 which bans commercial surrogacy," *The Times of India,* TNN, December 19, 2018, https://timesofindia.indiatimes.com/topic/Lok-Sabha-Passes-Surrogacy-(Regulation)-Bill-2016-Which-Bans-Commercial.

36. Sheela Saravanan, *A Transnational Feminist View of Surrogacy Biomarkets in India,* Singapore, Springer Nature Singapore Pte Ltd, 2018.

Chapter 2. Women's Issues

1. Martine Segalen, "Why there can be no such thing as 'ethical' surrogacy," *Travail, genre et sociétés*, vol. 2 (38), 2017, p. 54.

2. Céline Lemay, *La mise au monde, revisiter les savoirs*, Montréal, les Presses de l'Université de Montréal, 2017.

3. Maternity is a normal condition, not a disease, and women can experience healthy pregnancies and deliveries with no intervention necessary. There are risks, however, some of which are revealed only as the woman goes into labour. This explains why in the 1990s the World Health Organization (WHO) changed the name of the program aimed at reducing maternal mortality from "Safe Motherhood" to "Making Motherhood Safer."

4. Nathalie MacKinnon et al., "The Association Between Prenatal Stress and Externalizing Symptoms in Childhood: Evidence From the Avon Longitudinal Study of Parents and Children," *Biological Psychiatry*, vol. 83, Issue 2, January 15, 2018, p. 100-108.

5. Françoise Héritier, *Masculin/Féminin*, tome II, *Dissoudre la hiérarchie*, Paris, Éditions Odile Jacob, 2001, p. 22-23 [trans.].

6. Throughout history, women have been used to "produce" children that are then taken from them. This is well documented. But what is unprecedented is the social context surrounding the practice, which changes its meaning. Using a surrogate in the 21st century is like making a child on demand once a contract is drawn up; it no longer adheres to a social practice within a traditional culture.

7. Sylvie Martin, op. cit.

8. David Le Breton, "La question anthropologique de la gestation pour autrui," in Brigitte Feuillet-Liger and Maria-Claudia Crespo-Brauner (dir.), op. cit., p. 348 [trans.].

9. Elseline Hoekzema et al., "Pregnancy leads to long-lasting changes in human brain structure," *Nature Neuroscience*, 2017, 20, p. 287-296.

10. Laura Lange, "La gestation pour autrui. Quelles représentations du corps et de la volonté?" *Études*, vol. February, no. 2, 2014, p. 43-54, https://www.cairn.info/revue-etudes-2014-2-page-43.htm [trans.].

11. Association pour la santé publique du Québec (ASPQ), "Accoucher ou se faire accoucher," regional symposia on humanizing perinatal care, final report, *Bulletin de l'ASPQ,* vol. 5, no. 1, 1981, p. 5-16.

12. Some of the most prominent writers of the era include Ann Oakley, Barbara Ehrenreich, Adrienne Rich, and Sheila Kitzinger.

13. Ontario was the first province to legalize the midwifery practice (1994).

14. Andrée Rivard, *Histoire de l'accouchement dans un Québec moderne.* Montréal, Les éditions du remue-ménage, 2014, p. 349 [trans.].

15. ICIS data for 2016-2017: https://yourhealthsystem.cihi.ca/epub/search.jspa?href=https%3A//yourhealthsystem.cihi.ca/epub/SearchServlet.

16. Melinda Cooper and Catherine Waldby, *Clinical Labor: Tissue Donors and Research Subjects in the Global Bioeconomy,* Durham, Duke University Press, 2014, p. 84.

17. Ibid, p. 85.

18. Jennifer Lahl, "La vérité des grossesses à contrat," in Ana-Luna Stoicea-Deram, Marie-Josèphe Devillers et Catherine Morin Le Sech (coordination), *Pour le respect des femmes et des enfants, abolir la maternité de substitution,* TheBookEdition.com, 2019, p. 89-95.

19. Gènéthique, "Le principe constitutionnel de dignité à l'origine des lois de bioéthiques est-il en fin de vie?" May 17, 2018, http://www.genethique.org/fr/le-principe-constitutionnel-de-dignite-lorigine-des-lois-de-bioethiques-est-il-en-fin-de-vie-69725#.Wv4HokgvzIV [trans.].

20. Roxane Noel, "Commercial Surrogacy and Materialist Feminism," *What's wrong?* October 1, 2015, https://whatswrong-cvsp.com/2015/10/01/commercial-surrogacy-and-materialist-feminism/.

21. "L'enfantement pour autrui, esclavage des temps modernes," PDF Québec, 2017, http://www.pdfquebec.org/index_actualites.php#Brochure_GPA.

Uncorrected Galleys

22. Laura Harrison, "'I am the baby's real mother': Reproductive tourism, race, and the transnational construction of kinship," *Women's Studies International Forum 47*, 2014, p.152.

23. Delphine Lance, "Mettre à distance la maternité. La gestation pour autrui en Ukraine et aux États-Unis," *Ethnologie française*, no. 167, 2017, p. 410 [trans.].

24. https://fertilityconsultants.ca/become-a-surrogate/, accessed February 2020.

25. Porter l'enfant d'un autre: incursion dans l'univers des mères porteuses, https://ici.radio-canada.ca/nouvelle/1097065/incursion-univers-meres-porteuses-fannie-olivier, April 28, 2018. See introduction and note 21 for more information about this company. Acting as intermediary between ova donors, surrogates, and commissioning parents, it appears to be positioning itself to be ready for the eventual legalization of commercial donation and surrogacy.

26. The authors of the television report cited in the above note could have their objectivity questioned, especially since it is such a contentious topic.

27. David Riendeau, "Mère porteuse deux fois," *Journal de Montréal,* June 3, 2018, https://www.journaldemontreal.com/2018/06/03/mere-porteuse-deux-fois, accessed November 2018.

28. Sally Howard, "US army wives: the most sought-after surrogates in the world," *The Telegraph*, May 7, 2015, https://www.telegraph.co.uk/women/mother-tongue/11583541/US-army-wives-the-most-sought-after-surrogates-in-the-world.html, accessed October 2018. A 2010 article on the subject addressed the same question: Habiba Nosheen and Hilke Schellmann, "The Most Wanted Surrogates in the World," *Glamour,* October 4, 2010, https://www.glamour.com/story/the-most-wanted-surrogates-in-the-world, accessed October 2018.

29. Sylvie Epelboin (Head of Unit on Assisted Reproductive Techniques, groupe hospitalier Bichat-Claude Bernard), "Gestation pour autrui: une assistance médicale à la procréation comme les autres ?," *L'information psychiatrique*, vol. 87, no. 7, Paris, 2011, p. 578.

30. Ibid, p. 577.

31. HRC, op. cit., article 72, p. 17.

32. Alain Roy (pres.), *Pour un droit de la famille adapté aux nouvelles réalités conjugales et familiales,* Quebec, Comité consultatif sur le droit de la famille, Ministère de la justice du Québec, 2015, https://www.justice.gouv.qc.ca [trans.].

33. To be addressed in chapter 4.

34. WHO, "10 facts on breastfeeding," 2017, https://www.who.int/features/factfiles/breastfeeding/en/, viewed October 2018; Stanley Ip et al., "Breastfeeding and maternal and infant health outcomes in developed countries," *Evidence report/technology assessment,* no. 153, 2007, p. 1-186.

35. Lauren M. Papp, "Longitudinal Associations Between Breastfeeding and Observed Mother-Child Interaction Qualities in Early Childhood," *Child Care Health Development,* vol. 40, no. 5, 2014, p. 740-746.

36. Jérôme Courduriès, "La gestation pour autrui, faire naître des pères et des mères," in Isabelle Côté et al., op. cit., p. 138 [trans.].

37. Ibid.

38. Julie Bindel, "An Example of Capitalism Literally Milking the Poor," *Truthdig,* , April 19, 2017, https://www.truthdig.com/articles/an-example-of-capitalism-literally-milking-the-poor/.

39. Delphine Lance, op. cit., p. 416 [trans].

40. Ibid, p. 417 [trans.].

Chapter 3. The Child at the Heart of Surrogacy

1. A recent volume on surrogacy claims to distinguish itself by focusing on the "persons who are directly concerned." There is no mention of the child, who is undoubtedly concerned: "Contributions from a variety of socio-legal and cultural contexts address different perspectives on surrogacy, whether it is the experience of surrogate mothers, intended parents, and medical or legal intermediaries involved in some capacity with the surrogacy project." Isabelle Côté et al., op. cit., p. 11. [trans.].

2. On July 6, 2016, Justice Viviane Primeau permitted a biological father's common-law male partner to adopt twin girls born in 2012 to a surrogate mother in India, arguing that "the surrogacy debate should not punish the children (165) and that the Court is not responsible for addressing the wider debate on surrogacy motherhood (166)." Adoption-1631 2016 QCCQ 6872. Justice Primeau cited article 3 of the United Nations' Convention on the Rights of the Child. We will come back to this.

3. Claudine Brunetti-Pons et al., *Le "droit à l'enfant" et la filiation en France et dans le monde, Rapport final,* CEJESCO de l'Université de Reims, Mission de recherche droit et justice, Conformément à la Convention de recherche no 14.19, January 5, 2014 – January 5, 2017, p. 30. [trans.].

4. Sylvie Epelboin, op. cit., p. 577 [trans.].

5. Myriam Szejer and Jean-Pierre Winter, "Les maternités de substitution," in Jacques Besson and Mireille Galtier, *Que sont parents et bébés devenus?* ERES, "Les Dossiers de Spirale," 2010, p. 97-110 [trans.].

6. *Big Fertility,* by Jennifer Lahl, released in 2018 and available at https://vimeo.com/ondemand/bigfertility.

7. In the original French version, the word abandon was used as "(aban)don" to highlight the misuse of the term "don" which means "gift".

8. Sylvie Epelboin, op. cit., p. 577 [trans.].

9. Myriam Szejer and Jean-Pierre Winter, op. cit., p. 36 [trans.].

10. Martine Gross, "Pères gays et gestatrices," in Isabelle Côté et al., op. cit., p. 76 [trans.].

11. Ibid, p. 81.

12. Françoise Furkel, "L'incidence de la biomédecine sur la parenté ou le triomphe de l'amour de la vérité biologique," in Brigitte Feuillet-Liger and Maria-Claudia Crespo-Brauner (dir.). op. cit., p. 28.

13. Frequently cited studies by Susan Golombok et al. involve a very small sample size of children fourteen and under, as the

authors themselves point out: "Children born through reproductive donation: a longitudinal study of psychological adjustment," *Journal of Child Psychology and Psychiatry,* vol. 54, no. 6, 2013, p. 653-660; "A Longitudinal Study of Families Formed Through Reproductive Donation: Parent-Adolescent Relationships and Adolescent Adjustment at Age 14," *Developmental Psychology,* vol. 53, no. 10, 2017, p. 1966-1977.

14. Interview aired on *Dessine-moi un dimanche* with Franco Nuovo, Radio-Canada Première, September 16, 2018. The show's website describes the song as the "standout track from her recent album, *The Ballad of the Runaway Girl,* that [Isaac] describes as a love song to her biological mother, a quest for answers she has carried in her for years," https://ici.radio-canada.ca/premiere/emissions/dessine-moi-un-dimanche/segments/chronique/87201/elisapie-album-runaway-girl-mere-biologique.

15. Elisapie Issac in an interview with Sylvain Cormier, "Le chemin jusqu'à Elisapie," *Le Devoir, Le D magazine,* September 15-16, 2018, p. 9.

16. Convention on the Rights of the Child, Office of the High Commissioner, United Nations Human Rights, 1990, http://www.ohchr.org/EN/ProfessionalInterest/Pages/CRC.aspx.

17. Office of the High Commissioner, United Nations Human Rights, *Optional Protocol to the Convention on the Rights of the Child on the sale of children, child prostitution and child pornography,* article 2, 2000, https://www.ohchr.org/EN/ProfessionalInterest/Pages/OPSCCRC.aspx.

18. The report refers here to John W. Tobin, "To prohibit or permit: what is the (human) rights response to the practice of international commercial surrogacy?" *International and Comparative Law Quarterly,* vol. 63, no. 2, University of Melbourne Legal Studies research paper no. 689, 2014, p. 18-21 and 24-27, accessible at https://papers.ssrn.com/sol3/papers.cfm?abstract_id=2476751.

19. HRC, op. cit., article 35, p. 10-11.

20. Ibid, article 25, p. 7-8.

21. Ibid, article 64, p. 15-16.

22. Claire Ashmad, "The year international surrogacy came to the fore," *The Conversation*, December 25, 2014, https://theconversation.com/2014-the-year-international-surrogacy-came-to-the-fore-35495, accessed September 2018.

23. HRC, op. cit., p. 8.

24. David Le Breton, op. cit., p. 348 [trans.].

Chapter 4. Wanting a Child versus Human Dignity

1. HRC, op. cit.

2. http://mafr.fr/search/?q=GPA.

3. Adeline A. Allen, "Surrogacy and Limitations to Freedom of Contract: Toward Being more Fully Human," *Harvard Journal of Law and Public Policy*, vol. 41, no. 3, 2018, p. 806-807; (a) Debora L. Spar, The Baby Business: How Money, Science, and Politics Drive the Commerce of Conception, Harvard Business School Press.: Boston, Massachusetts, 2006, p. 93.

4. Ibid.

5. Francis Kernaleguen, "Les incidences de la biomédecine sur la parenté en droit français: reconsidérer la parenté," in Brigitte Feuillet-Liger and Maria-Claudia Crespo-Brauner (dir.), op. cit., p. 108 [trans.].

6. Héritier, Françoise, op. cit., 1996, p. 260 [trans.].

7. David Le Breton, op. cit., p. 348 [trans.].

8. Peter Conrad, *The medicalization of society: on the transformation of human conditions into treatable disorders*, Baltimore, Johns Hopkins University Press, 2007. Conrad is one of the biggest names in this field of research.

9. Assisted Human Reproduction Canada, *Your guide to infertility and assisted human reproduction (AHR)*, Ottawa, Government of Canada, 2012, http://publications.gc.ca/collections/collection_2011/pac-ahrc/H179-4-2010-eng.pdf.

10. Association des gynécologues et obstétriciens du Québec, keyword: infertility: http://www.gynecoquebec.com/en/woman-health/gynecology/20-infertility.html, accessed March 2020.

11. Government of Canada, https://www.canada.ca/en/public-health/services/fertility/fertility.html, accessed October 2018.

12. Laura Harrison, op. cit.

13. This means that pregnancy by proxy is not a medical treatment: Claudine Brunetti-Pons et al., op. cit., p. 30 [trans.].

14. Ibid, p. 377 [trans.].

15. Myriam Szejer and Jean-Pierre Winter, op. cit., p. 35 [trans.].

16. Martine Segalen, op. cit., p. 56.

17. Françoise Héritier, 1996, op. cit., p. 284.

18. Jean-Mathias Sargologos, Sébastien de Crèvecoeur, and Jacques Duffourg-Muller, "En tant qu'homosexuels, il est de notre devoir de prendre position contre la PMA et la GPA," *Le Figaro,* January 26, 2018, http://www.lefigaro.fr/vox/societe/2018/01/26/31003-20180126ARTFIG00197-en-tant-qu-homosexuels-il-est-de-notre-devoir-de-prendre-position-contre-la-pma-et-la-gpa.php, accessed October 2018 [trans.].

19. Julie Bindel and Gary Powell, *Gay Rights and Surrogacy Wrongs: Say "No" to Wombs-for-Rent,* 2018, http://www.stopsurrogacynow.com/gay-rights-and-surrogacy-wrongs-say-no-to-wombs-for-rent/#sthash.JOFdejfl.dpbs, accessed November 2018.

20. The Indian Council of Medical Research has also noted a correlation between the decrease in adoption and increase in births to surrogate mothers. Sheela Saravanan, *A Transnational Feminist View of Surrogacy Biomarkets in India,* op. cit., p. 96.

21. Jean-François Chicoine, "La politique du vêlage," *La Presse* +, April 12, 2018, https://plus.lapresse.ca/screens/f49d9bc9-c3d9-4f38-b7a2-f37f9de73470__7C___o.html, accessed October 2018 [trans.].

22. Sylvie Epelboin, op. cit., p. 574 [trans.].

23. Ibid, p. 365 [trans.].

24. Sylviane Agasinski, *Corps en miettes,* Paris, Flammarion, 2013, p. 17 [trans.].

25. Agnès Gruda, "Ventres à louer: Voyage au coeur d'une 'usine à bébés'," *La Presse* +, October 18, 2014, https://www.lapresse.ca/

Uncorrected Galleys

international/asie-oceanie/201410/18/01-10456-ventres-a-louer-en-inde.php, accessed October 2018 [trans.].

26. Françoise Dekeuwer-Défossez, op. cit., p. 367 [trans.].

Chapter 5. The Pieces of the Puzzle

1. Irene Woo et al., "Perinatal outcomes after natural conception versus in vitro fertilization (IVF) in gestational surrogates: a model to evaluate IVF treatment versus maternal effects," *Fertility and Sterility*, vol. 108, no. 6, 2017, p. 993-998.

2. Yona Nicolau, "Outcomes of surrogate pregnancies in California and hospital economics of surrogate maternity and newborn care," *World Journal of Obstetrics and Gynecology*, vol. 10, no. 4, 2015, p. 102-107.

3. https://www.pregnancyinfo.ca/birth/delivery/caesarean-section/, accessed October 2018.

4. Sheela Saravanan, *A Transnational Feminist View of Surrogacy Biomarkets in India*, op. cit., p. 84.

5. https://surrogacy360.org/relationship/children/, accessed October 2018.

6. https://surrogacy360.org/relationship/surrogates/, accessed October 2018.

7. Michael Cook, "Idaho surrogate mother dies from pregnancy complications," *BioEdge*, October 17, 2015, https://www.bioedge.org/bioethics/idaho-surrogate-mother-dies-from-pregnancy-complications/11614, accessed January 2019.

8. https://www.cnn.com/2020/01/20/us/surrogate-mom-dies-trnd/index.html, accessed February 2020.

9. Sarah Jacob-Wagner, "L'état des connaissances sur les expériences des femmes qui choisissent de porter un enfant pour autrui," in Isabelle Côté et al., op. cit., p. 146-165.

10. Godelier, M. op. cit., p. 370 [trans.].

11. Martine Segalen, op. cit., p. 57-58.

12. Comité consultatif sur le droit de la famille, op. cit., p. 170 [trans.].

13. Ibid.

14. Ibid.

15. I forwarded comments to Health Canada on December 19, 2018 entitled "Règlement sur le remboursement relatif à la procréation assistée: un choix politique qui favorise l'industrie de la PA ?" ("*Reimbursement Related to Assisted Human Reproduction Regulations: a political choice favouring the AHR industry*?").

Conclusion

1. Comité consultatif sur le droit de la famille, op. cit., p. 170 [trans.].

2. David M. Smolin, "The One Hundred Thousand Dollar Baby: The Ideological Roots of a New American Export," *Cumberland Law Review*, vol. 49, no. 1, 2018, p. 1-54.

Uncorrected Galleys

References

Assisted Human Reproduction Act, S.C. 2004, c. 2.

Act to amend the Civil Code and other legislative provisions concerning adoption and the disclosure of information, SQ 2017, c 12.

Agasinski, Sylviane, *Corps en miettes*, Paris, Flammarion, 2013.

Assisted Human Reproduction Canada, *Your guide to infertility and assisted human reproduction (AHR)*, Ottawa, Government of Canada, 2012, http://publications.gc.ca/collections/collection_2011/pac-ahrc/H179-4-2010-eng.pdf.

Association des obstétriciens et gynécologues du Québec, keyword: infertility: http://www.gynecoquebec.com/en/woman-health/gynecology/20-infertility.html, accessed March 2020.

Association pour la santé publique du Québec, "Accoucher ou se faire accoucher," colloques régionaux sur l'humanisation des soins en périnatalié, rapport-synthèse, *Bulletin de l'ASPQ*, vol. 5, no 1, 1981, p. 5-16.

Allen, Adeline A., "Surrogacy and Limitations to Freedom of Contract: Toward Being More Fully Human," *Harvard Journal of Law and Public Policy*, vol. 41, no 3, 2018, p. 753-811.

Ashmad, Claire, "The year international surrogacy came to the fore," *The Conversation*, December 25, 2014, https://theconversation.com/2014-the-year-international-surrogacy-came-to-the-fore-35495, accessed September 2018.

Barry, Laurent S. *et al.*, *Glossaire de la parenté*, *L'HOMME*, 154-155, 2000, p. 721-732, https://journals.openedition.org/lhomme/58.

Beeson, Diane, Darnovsky, Marcy et Abby Lippman, "What's in a name? Variations in terminology of third-party reproduction," *Reproductive BioMedicine Online*, 2015, p. 805–814.

Bindel, Julie, "An Example of Capitalism Literally Milking the Poor," *Thruthdig*, 19 avril 2017, https://www.truthdig.com/articles/an-example-of-capitalism-literally-milking-the-poor/, accessed May 2017.

Bindel, Julie and Gary Powell, *Gay Rights and Surrogacy Wrongs: Say "No" to Wombs-for-Rent*, 2018, http://www.stopsurrogacy-now.com/gay-rights-and-surrogacy-wrongs-say-no-to-wombs-for-rent/#sthash.JOFdejfl.dpbs, accessed November 2018.

Brunetti-Pons, Claudine *et al.*, *Le "droit à l'enfant" et la filiation en France et dans le monde, Rapport final*, CEJESCO de l'Université de Reims, Mission de recherche droit et justice, Conformément à la Convention de recherche n° 14.19, 5 janvier 2015 - 5 janvier 2017.

Cambodia-police raid child surrogacy ring involving 33 surrogate mothers, July 23, 2018, Génèthique, http://www.genethique.org/en/cambodia-police-raid-child-surrogacy-ring-involving-33-surrogate-mothers-70121.html#.Xl7kCErCo2w.

Canadian Institute for Health Information (CIHI), Health Indicators Interactive Tools, https://yourhealthsystem.cihi.ca/epub/search.jspa?href=https%3A//yourhealthsystem.cihi.ca/epub/SearchServlet.

Chicoine, Jean-François, "La politique du vêlage," *La Presse +*, 12 avril 2018, http://plus.lapresse.ca/screens/f49d9bc9-c3d9-4f38-b7a2-f37f9de734707C0.html.

Civil Code of Quebec, CQLR c CCQ-1991, c. 64, art 541, as amended by SQ 2002, c. 6, s 30.

Comité consultatif sur le droit de la famille, ministère de la Justice du Québec, Alain Roy (prés.), *Pour un droit de la famille adapté aux nouvelles réalités conjugales et familiales*, Québec, 2015, https://www.justice.gouv.qc.ca.

Conrad, Peter, *The medicalization of society: on the transformation of human conditions into treatable disorders*, Baltimore, John Hopkins University Press, 2007.

Convention on the Rights of the Child, Office of the High Commissioner, United Nations Human Rights, 1990, http://www.ohchr.org/EN/ProfessionalInterest/Pages/CRC.aspx.

Cook, Michael, "Idaho surrogate mother dies from pregnancy complication," *BioEdge*, 17 octobre 2015, https://www.bioedge.org/bioethics/idaho-surrogate-mother-dies-from-pregnancy-complications/11614.

Cooper, Melinda et Catherine Waldby, *Clinical Labor: Tissue Donors and Research Subjects in the Global Bioeconomy*, Durham, Duke University Press, 2014, p. 62-90.

Cormier, Sylvain, "Le chemin jusqu'à Elisapie," *Le Devoir, Le D magazine*, 15-16 septembre 2018, p. 9.

Côté, Isabelle, Lavoie, Kevin et Jérôme Courduriès (dir.), *Perspectives internationales sur la gestation pour autrui, Expériences des personnes concernées et contextes d'action*, Québec, Presses de l'Université du Québec, 2018.

Coulombe-Pontbriand, Myriam, "Maternité et liberté. Malaise du féminisme moderne," *Argument*, vol. 2, no 10, 2008, http://www.revueargument.ca/.

Courduriès, Jérôme, "Ce que fabrique la gestation pour autrui," *Journal des anthropologues*, 144-145, 2016, p. 53-76.

Courduriès, Jérôme, "La gestation pour autrui, faire naître des pères et des mères," dans Côté, Isabelle, Lavoie, Kevin et Jérôme Courduriès (dir.), *Perspectives internationales sur la*

Uncorrected Galleys

gestation pour autrui, Expériences des personnes concernées et contextes d'action, Québec, Presses de l'Université du Québec, 2018, p. 123-141.

Creative Family Connections.com, en ligne, https://www.creativefamilyconnections.com/us-surrogacy-law-map, accessed February 2020.

Cribb, Robert et Emma Jarratt, "How Canada is becoming a key player in global surrogacy," *The Star*, June 25, 2016, https://www.thestar.com/news/world/2016/06/25/how-canada-is-becoming-a-key-player-in-global-surrogacy.html.

de Beauvoir, Simone, *Le deuxième sexe*, Paris, Gallimard, 1970.

Déchaux, Jean-Hugues, "Les défis des nouvelles techniques de reproduction : comment la parenté entre en politique," dans Brigitte Feuillet-Liger, et Maria-Claudia Crespo-Brauner (dir.), *Les incidences de la biomédecine sur la parenté*, Bruxelles, Bruylant, 2014, p. 313-335.

Dekeuwer-Défossez, Françoise, "Réflexions conclusives," dans Brigitte Feuillet-Liger et Maria-Claudia Crespo-Brauner, (dir.), *Les incidences de la biomédecine sur la parenté*, Bruxelles, Bruylant, 2014, p. 360-367.

De Koninck, Maria, "Dévalorisation et déqualification du rôle maternel: est-ce la faute des féministes ?» Speech delivered at the symposium *Marcher sur des œufs – Certains enjeux du féminisme aujourd'hui,* organized by the Conseil du statut de la femme, 1998, https://www.csf.gouv.qc.ca/wp-content/uploads/allocution-de-maria-de-koninck-colloque-marcher-sur-des-oeufs.pdf.

Dib, Lina, "Un député veut décriminaliser les grossesses payées,» *Le Nouvelliste*, 27 mars 2018, https://www.lenouvelliste.ca/actualites/le-fil-groupe-capitales-medias/un-depute-veut-decriminaliser-les-grossesses-payees-0fc3785bbdf0f586b6e4d-71d46517e39.

Ekman, Kajsa Ekis, *Being and Being Bought: Prostitution, Surrogacy and the Split Self*, cité dans Catherine Lynch, "Ethical Case for Abolishing all Forms of Surrogacy," *SundayGuardianLive*, 28 octobre 2017, https://www.sundayguardianlive.com/lifestyle/11390-ethical-case-abolishing-all-forms-surrogacy.

Encyclopedia Universalis, online: https://www.universalis.fr/encyclopedie/.

Epelboin, Sylvie, "Gestation pour autrui : une assistance médicale à la procréation comme les autres ?," *L'information psychiatrique*, vol. 87, no7, Paris, 2011, p. 573-579.

Frison-Roche, Marie-Anne, "Prohibition de la GPA : convergence absolue entre droits des femmes et droits des enfants,» 2 May 2016, http://mafr.fr/fr/article/denoncer-la-strategie-des-industriels-de-lhumain-c/, accessed October 2018.

Furkel, Françoise, "L'incidence de la biomédecine sur la parenté ou le triomphe de l'amour de la vérité biologique," dans Brigitte Feuillet-Liger et Maria-Claudia Crespo-Brauner (dir.), *Les incidences de la biomédecine sur la parenté*, Bruxelles, Bruylant, 2014, p. 23-53.

Godelier, Maurice, "Systèmes de parenté et formes de famille," *Recherches de Science Religieuse*, tome 102, no 3, 2014, p. 357-372.

Golombok, Susan *et al.* "Children born through reproductive donation: a longitudinal study of psychological adjustment," *Journal of Child Psychology and Psychiatry*, vol. 54, no 6, 2013, p 653–660.

Golombok, Susan *et al.*, "A Longitudinal Study of Families Formed Through Reproductive Donation: Parent-Adolescent Relationships and Adolescent Adjustment at Age 14", *Developmental Psychology*, vol. 53, no 10, 2017, p. 1966–1977.

Government of Canada, https://www.canada.ca/en/public-health/services/fertility/fertility.html, accessed October 2018.

Gross, Martine, "Pères gays et gestatrices,» dans Côté, Isabelle, Lavoie, Kevin et Jérôme Courduriès (dir.), *Perspectives internationales sur la gestation pour autrui, Expériences des personnes concernées et contextes d'action*, Québec, Presses de l'Université du Québec, 2018, p.69-89.

Gruben, Vanessa, Cattapan, Alana and Angela Cameron (eds), *Surrogacy in Canada, Critical Perspectives in Law and Policy*, Toronto, Irwin Law, 2018.

Gruda, Agnès, "Ventres à louer: Voyage au cœur d'une 'usine à bébés'," *La Presse +*, 18 octobre 2014, https://www.lapresse.ca/international/asie-oceanie/201410/18/01-4810456-ventres-a-louer-en-inde.php.

Habiba, Nosheenm and Hilke Schellmann, "The Most Wanted Surrogates in the World," *Glamour*, 4 October 2010, https://www.glamour.com/story/the-most-wanted-surrogates-in-the-world.

Harrison, Laura, "'I am the baby's real mother': Reproductive tourism, race, and the transnational construction of kinship," *Women's Studies International Forum 47*, 2014, p. 145-156.

Héritier, Françoise, *Les deux sœurs et leur mère. Anthropologie de l'inceste*, Paris, Odile Jacob, 1994.

Héritier, Françoise, *Masculin/Féminin*, tome I, *La pensée de la différence*, Paris, Éditions Odile Jacob, 1996.

Héritier, Françoise, *Masculin/Féminin*, tome II, *Dissoudre la hiérarchie*, Paris, Éditions Odile Jacob, 2001.

Héritier, Françoise, "La filiation, état social," *La revue lacanienne*, vol. 3 no 8, 2010, p. 33-36.

Hoekzema, Elseline *et al*, "Pregnancy leads to long-lasting changes in human brain structure," *Nature Neuroscience*, 2017, 20, p. 287-296.

Houle, Gilles et Roch Hurtubise, "Parler de faire des enfants, une question vitale," *Recherches sociographiques*, vol. 32, n° 3, 1991, p. 385-414.

Howard, Sally, "US army wives: the most sought-after surrogates in the world," *The Telegraph*, 7 May 2015, https://www.telegraph.co.uk/women/mother-tongue/11583541/US-army-wives-the-most-sought-after-surrogates-in-the-world.html.

Human Rights Council (HRC), *Report of the Special Rapporteur on the sale and sexual exploitation of children, including child prostitution, child pornography and other child sexual abuse material*, 37th session, February 26 – March 23, (A/HRC/37/60), https://ap.ohchr.org/documents/dpage_e.aspx?m=102 accessed February 2020.

Iacub, Marcela, *L'empire du ventre. Pour une autre histoire de la maternité*, Paris, Fayard, 2004.

Inhorn, Marcia C., "Women, Consider Freezing your Eggs," *CNN. com*, 2013, https ://www.cnn.com/2013/04/09/opinion/inhorn-egg-freezing/index.html.

Institut de la statistique du Québec, en ligne: http://www.stat.gouv.qc.ca/statistiques/.

Ip, Stanley *et al.*, "Breastfeeding and maternal and infant health outcomes in developed countries," *Evidence report/technology assessment*, no 153, 2007, p. 1–186.

Jacob-Wagner, Sarah, "L'état des connaissances sur les expériences des femmes qui choisissent de porter un enfant pour autrui," dans Côté, Isabelle, Lavoie, Kevin et Jérôme Courduriès (dir.), *Perspectives internationales sur la gestation pour autrui, Expériences des personnes concernées et contextes d'action*, Québec, Presses de l'Université du Québec, 2018, p. 146-165.

Joyal, Renée, "Parenté, parentalité et filiation. Des questions cruciales pour l'avenir de nos enfants et de nos sociétés," *Enfances, familles, générations*. Évolution des normes juridiques et nouvelles formes de régulation de la famille : regards croisés sur le couple et l'enfant, Renée Joyal et Alain Roy (dir.), n° 5, 2006, p. 1-16.

Uncorrected Galleys

Kernaleguen, Francis, "Les incidences de la biomédecine sur la parenté en droit français: reconsidérer la parenté," dans Brigitte Feuillet-Liger et Maria-Claudia Crespo-Brauner (dir.), *Les incidences de la biomédecine sur la parenté*, Bruxelles, Bruylant, 2014, p. 107-123.

Lafontaine, Céline, *Le corps marché, La marchandisation de la vie humaine à l'ère de la bioéconomie*, Paris, Seuil, 2014.

Lahl, Jennifer, "La vérité des grossesses à contrat," in Ana-Luna Stoicea-Deram, Marie-Josèphe Devillers et Catherine Morin Le Sech, (coordination), *Pour le respect des femmes et des enfants, abolir la maternité de substitution*, TheBookEdition.com, 2019, p. 89-95.

Lance, Delphine, "Mettre à distance la maternité. La gestation pour autrui en Ukraine et aux États-Unis," *Ethnologie française*, n° 167, 2017, p. 410.

Lange, Laura, "La gestation pour autrui. Quelles représentations du corps et de la volonté?," *Études*, vol. février, n° 2, 2014, p. 43-54, https://www.cairn.info/revue-etudes-2014-2-page-43.htm.

Le Breton, David, "La question anthropologique de la gestation pour autrui," dans Brigitte Feuillet-Liger et Maria-Claudia Crespo-Brauner (dir.), *Les incidences de la biomédecine sur la parenté*, Bruxelles, Bruylant, 2014, p. 337-348.

Lemay, Céline, *La mise au monde, revisiter les savoirs*, Montréal, les Presses de l'Université de Montréal, 2017.

"Le principe constitutionnel de dignité à l'origine des lois de bioéthiques est-il en fin de vie?," *Gènéthique*, 17 mai 2018, http://www.genethique.org/fr/le-principe-constitutionnel-de-dignite-lorigine-des-lois-de-bioethiques-est-il-en-fin-de-vie-69725#.Wv4HokgvzIV.

"Lok Sabha passes Surrogacy (Regulation) Bill 2016 which bans commercial surrogacy," *The Times of India*, TNN, December 19, 2018, https://timesofindia.indiatimes.com/topic/

Lok-Sabha-Passes-Surrogacy-(Regulation)-Bill-2016-Which-Bans-Commercial

MacKinnon, Nathalie *et al.*, "The Association Between Prenatal Stress and Externalizing Symptoms in Childhood: Evidence from The Avon Longitudinal Study of Parents and Children," *Biological Psychiatry*, vol. 83, no 2, 15 January 2018, p. 100-108.

Martin, Sylvie, *Le désenfantement du monde*, Montréal, Liber, 2011.

Motluk, Alison, "After pleading guilty for paying surrogates, business is booming for this fertility matchmaker," *The Globe and Mail*, 28 February 2016, https://www.theglobeandmail.com/life/health-and-fitness/health/business-is-booming-for-fertility-matchmaker-leia-swanberg/article28930242/.

Nicolau, Yona, "Outcomes of surrogate pregnancies in California and hospital economics of surrogate maternity and newborn care," *World Journal of Obstetrics and Gynecology*, vol. 10, no 4, 2015, p. 102-107.

"Nigeria police raid Lagos 'baby factory'," *BBC News in Africa*, 30 September 2019, https://www.bbc.com/news/world-africa-49877287.

Noel, Roxane, "Commercial Surrogacy and Materialist Feminism," *What's wrong?*, October 1, 2015, https://whatswrongcvsp.com/2015/10/01/commercial-surrogacy-and-materialist-feminism/.

Office of the High Commissioner, United Nations Human Rights, *Optional Protocol to the Convention on the Rights of the Child on the sale of children, child prostitution and child pornography*, 2000, https://www.ohchr.org/EN/ProfessionalInterest/Pages/OPSCCRC.aspx

Papp, Lauren M., "Longitudinal Associations Between Breastfeeding and Observed Mother-Child Interaction Qualities in

Early Childhood," *Child Care Health Development*, vol. 40, no 5, 2014, p. 740-746.

PDF Québec, "L'enfantement pour autrui, esclavage des temps modernes," 2017, http://www.pdfquebec.org/index_actualites. php#Brochure_GPA.

Porqueres i Gené, Enric, "Corps relationnel, inceste et parenté aux temps de la génétique globalisée," *Ethnologie française*, n° 167, 2017, p. 519-530.

Riendeau, David, "Mère porteuse deux fois,» *Journal de Montréal*, 3 juin 2018, https://www.journaldemontreal.com/2018/06/03/ mere-porteuse-deux-fois.

Rivard, Andrée, *Histoire de l'accouchement dans un Québec moderne*. Montréal, Les éditions du remue-ménage, 2014, p. 349.

Rossignol, Michel, Boughrassa, Faiza et Jean-Marie Moutquin, "Mesures prometteuses pour diminuer le recours aux interventions obstétricales évitables pour les femmes à faible risqué," *Avis de l'INESSS*, ETMIS, 2012, p. 1-134.

Saravanan, Sheela, "An ethnomethodological approach to examine exploitation in the context of capacity, trust and experience of commercial surrogacy in India," *Philosophy, Ethics and Humanities in Medicine*, 2013, 8:10, https://peh-med.biomedcentral.com/articles/10.1186/1747-5341-8-10.

Saravanan, Sheela, *A Transnational Feminist View of Surrogacy Biomarkets in India*, Singapour, Springer Nature Singapore Pte Ltd, 2018.

Sargologos, Jean-Mathias, de Crèvecoeur, Sébastien et Jacques Duffourg-Muller, "En tant qu'homosexuels, il est de notre devoir de prendre position contre la PMA et la GPA," *Le Figaro*, 26 janvier 2018, http://www.lefigaro.fr/vox/societe/ 2018/01/26/31003-20180126ARTFIG00197-en-tant-qu-homosexuels-il-est-de-notre-devoir-de-prendre-position-contre-la-pma-et-la-gpa.php.

Scott, Joan W., "Gender: A Useful Category of Historical Analysis," *The American Historical Review*, vol. 91, no 5, 1988, p. 1053–1075.

Segalen, Martine, "Why there can be no such thing as 'ethical' surrogacy," *Travail, genre et sociétés*, Vol. 2 (38), 2017, p. 53-73.

Slavery Convention (UN), https://www.ohchr.org/EN/Professional Interest/Pages/SlaveryConvention.aspx.

Smolin, David M., "The One Hundred Thousand Dollar Baby: The Ideological Roots of a New American Export," *Cumberland Law Review*, vol. 49, no. 1, 2018, p. 1-54.

South-East Asia, a real reproduction supply chain for Chinese couples, July 12, 2018, Gènéthique, http://www.genethique.org/en/south-east-asia-real-reproduction-supply-chain-chinese-couples-70069.html#.Xl7GnErCo2w.

Statistics Canada, online, http://www23.statcan.gc.ca/imdb/p3Var.pl?Function=DEC&Id=410445.

Surrogacy360.org, online, https://surrogacy360.org/considering-surrogacy/current-law/

Szejer, Myriam et Jean-Pierre Winter, "Les maternités de substitution," dans Jacques Besson et Mireille Galtier, *Que sont parents et bébés devenus?* ERES, "Les Dossiers de Spirale," 2010, p. 97-110.

Testart, Jacques, *Faire des enfants demain*, Paris, Seuil, 2014.

Tobin, John W., "To prohibit or permit: what is the (human) rights response to the practice of international commercial surrogacy?," *International and Comparative Law Quarterly*, vol. 63, no 2, University of Melbourne Legal Studies research paper no 689, 2014, https://papers.ssrn.com/sol3/papers.cfm?abstract_id=2476751.

World Health Organization, online, https://www.who.int/home.

Uncorrected Galleys

Woo, Irene *et al.*, "Perinatal outcomes after natural conception versus in vitro fertilization (IVF) in gestational surrogates: a model to evaluate IVF treatment versus maternal effects", *Fertility and Sterility*, vol. 108, no 6, 2017, p. 993-998. https://peh-med.biomedcentral.com/articles/10.1186/1747-5341-8-10.

ALSO FROM BARAKA BOOKS

Still Crying for Help
The Failure of our Mental Health Services
Sadia Messaili

Through the Mill
Girls and Women in the Quebec Cotton Textile Industry, 1881-1951
Gail Cuthbert Brandt

Storming the Old Boys' Citadel
Two Pioneer Women Architects of 19th Century North America
Carla Blank and Tania Martin

The Question of Separatism, Quebec and the Struggle Over Sovereignty
Jane Jacobs

A Distinct Alien Race, The Untold Story of Franco-Americans
David Vermette

The Einstein File, The FBI's Secret War
on the World's Most Famous Scientist
Fred Jerome

Montreal, City of Secrets, Confederate Operations in Montreal
During the American Civil War
Barry Sheehy

Washington's Long War on Syria
Stephen Gowans

FICTION

Yasmeen Haddad Loves Joanasi Maqaittik
Carolyn Marie Souaid

Exile Blues, A Novel
Douglas Gary Freeman

Fog, A Novel
Rana Bose

Things Worth Burying
Matt Mayr

Uncorrected Galleys

Uncorrected Galleys